Usui Tibetan Reiki Healing Energy Master / Teacher Student Manual

Text Copyright 2016 Mark A. Ashford Consulting Inc.
All Rights Reserved
Paperback: 978-1-988441-50-4
eBook: 978-1-990876-77-6

Usui Tibetan Reiki Healing Energy Master / Teacher Student Manual

This is the Student Manual for Usui Tibetan Reiki Healing Energy IV – Master / Teacher. It is available as either a physical book, eBook or Audio Book. The material provides additional information and helps in exploring Reiki and is a refence for your life connection with this pure, universal energy.

There are three reasons to be attuned to Usui Tibetan Reiki Healing Energy!

1. Attuning yourself to Reiki energy has a beneficial and mindful effect on you spiritually.
2. Attunement allows you to connect to healing energy when you need it.
3. Attunement gives you the knowledge and ability to connect with healing energy not only for yourself, but others in your family and friends.

This book is designed for self-study and to support understanding of this level of Usui Tibetan Reiki healing energy.

The cost of the course includes:

1. A period of your own self-paced study.
2. A certificate of completion.

For blog posts, courses, and to book a personal remote session in Usui Tibetan Reiki Healing, or, to connect with Mark for an information session, visit Mark's website: https://www.markaashford.com and click on Contact.

Mark A. Ashford
Usui Tibetan Reiki Master and Teacher
information@markaashford.com

Usui Tibetan Reiki Healing Energy Master / Teacher Student Manual

1 TABLE OF TABLES 8

DR. USUI'S CONCEPTS AND FIVE PRINCIPLES 9

   1.1 KANJI 9
   1.2 ENGLISH 9

2 SUGGESTIONS FOR TEACHING 11

3 REIKI MASTER MANTRA 12

4 MICHAEL'S SWORD TECHNIQUE 13

   4.1 DISASSOCIATED MEMORY 13
   4.2 ASSOCIATED CONSCIOUS MEMORY 13
   4.3 TISSUE OR NEUROMUSCULAR MEMORY 13

5 PREPARATION 14

   5.1 HELPING THE CLIENT UNDERSTAND 16

6 TREE OF LIFE MEDITATION 18

7 CHAKRAS INVOCATION – FIRST TIME INVOCATION FOR CHAKRAS 19

8 SECOND TIME INVOCATION FOR CHAKRAS 20

9 GROUNDING MEDITATION 21

10 THE USUI SYSTEM OF ATTUNEMENTS 22

   10.1 REIKI I – INITIATORY ATTUNEMENT 22
   10.2 ATTUNEMENT #1 OF 4 22
   10.2.1 PART ONE 22
   10.2.2 PART 2 23
   10.2.3 PART 3 23
   10.3 ATTUNEMENT #2 OF 4 24
   10.3.1 PART 2 24
   10.4 PART 3 24
   10.5 ATTUNEMENT #3 OF 4 25
   10.5.1 PART ONE 25
   10.5.2 PART 2 25
   10.5.3 PART THREE 26
   10.6 ATTUNEMENT #4 OF 4 26

Usui Tibetan Reiki Healing Energy Master / Teacher Student Manual

- 10.6.1 PART ONE 26
- 10.6.2 PART 2 27
- 10.6.3 PART 3 27

11 REIKI II—INITIATORY ATTUNEMENT 28

- 11.1 PART ONE 28
- 11.1.1 PART 2 29
- 11.1.2 PART 3 29
- 11.2 REIKI III—MASTER/TEACHER INITIATORY ATTUNEMENT 30
- 11.2.1 PART ONE 30
- 11.3 PART 2 30
- 11.4 PART 3 31
- 11.5 PART 4 31

12 REIKI LEVEL I INITIATORY ATTUNEMENT USUI/TIBETAN METHOD 31

- 12.1 ATTUNEMENT #1 OF 4 32
- 12.1.1 PREPARING THE STUDENT FOR ATTUNEMENT 32
- 12.1.2 PART ONE 32
- 12.1.3 PART 2—STAND IN FRONT OF STUDENT 33
- 12.1.4 PART THREE—STAND BEHIND STUDENT 33
- 12.1.5 PART 4—STAND IN FRONT OF THE STUDENT 34
- 12.2 ATTUNEMENT #2 OF 4 34
- 12.2.1 PREPARING THE STUDENT FOR THE ATTUNEMENT 34
- PART ONE 35
- 12.2.2 PART 2—STAND IN FRONT OF STUDENT 35
- 12.2.3 PART THREE—STAND BEHIND THE STUDENT 36
- 12.2.4 PART 4—STAND IN FRONT OF STUDENTS 36
- 12.3 ATTUNEMENT 3 OF 4 36
- 12.3.1 PREPARING THE STUDENT FOR ATTUNEMENT 37
- 12.3.2 PART ONE—STAND BEHIND STUDENT 37
- 12.3.3 PART 2—STAND IN FRONT OF STUDENTS 38
- 12.3.4 PART THREE—STAND BEHIND THE STUDENT 38
- 12.3.5 PART 4—STAND IN FRONT OF THE STUDENT 39
- 12.4 ATTUNEMENT 4 OF 4 39
- 12.4.1 PREPARING THE STUDENT FOR ATTUNEMENT 39
- 12.4.2 PART ONE—STAND BEHIND STUDENT 40
- 12.4.3 PART 2—STAND IN FRONT OF STUDENTS 40
- 12.4.4 PART THREE—STAND BEHIND THE STUDENT 41
- 12.4.5 PART 4—STAND IN FRONT OF THE STUDENT 41

13 REIKI LEVEL II INITIATORY ATTUNEMENT USUI/TIBETAN METHOD 42

- 13.1 PREPARING YOURSELF AND THE ROOM FOR THE ATTUNEMENT PROCESS 42
- 13.1.1 PREPARING THE STUDENT FOR ATTUNEMENT 42
- 13.1.2 PART ONE—STAND BEHIND THE STUDENT 42
- 13.1.3 PART 2—STAND IN FRONT OF STUDENT 43

13.1.4	PART THREE—STAND BEHIND THE STUDENT	44
13.1.5	PART 4—STAND IN FRONT OF THE STUDENT	44

14 REIKI LEVEL III INITIATORY ATTUNEMENT USUI/TIBETAN METHOD ... 45

14.1	PART ONE	45
14.1.1	PART 2—STAND IN FRONT OF STUDENT	46
14.1.2	PART THREE—STAND BEHIND THE STUDENT	46
14.1.3	PART 4—STAND IN FRONT OF THE STUDENT	47

15 REIKI MASTER/TEACHER ATTUNEMENT USUI/TIBETAN METHOD ... 48

15.1	PREPARING YOURSELF AND THE ROOM FOR THE ATTUNEMENT PROCESS	48
15.1.1	PREPARING THE STUDENT FOR ATTUNEMENT	48
15.1.2	PART ONE	48
15.1.3	PART 2—STAND IN FRONT OF STUDENT	49
15.1.4	PART THREE—STAND BEHIND THE STUDENT	50
15.1.5	PART 4—STAND IN FRONT OF STUDENTS	50

16 WATER CEREMONY AND MEDITATION—MASTER/TEACHER ATTUNEMENT ... 51

16.1	OPTIONAL MEDITATION FOR MASTER/TEACHER ATTUNEMENT	51
16.2	WATER CEREMONY OPTIONAL FOR REIKI MASTER/TEACHER ATTUNEMENT	51

17 USUI REIKI LEVEL I TEACHING NOTES ... 53

18 USUI REIKI LEVEL II TEACHING NOTES ... 54

19 USUI REIKI LEVEL III TEACHING NOTES ... 55

20 USUI/TIBETAN REIKI MASTER/TEACHER TEACHING NOTES ... 56

21 ATTUNEMENT GUIDE ... 58

21.1	REIKI LEVEL I ATTUNEMENT USUI/TIBETAN METHOD	58
21.2	ATTUNEMENT 1/4	58
21.3	ATTUNEMENT 2/4	58
21.4	ATTUNEMENT	59
21.5	ATTUNEMENT 4/4	60

22 REIKI LEVEL II ATTUNEMENT USUI/TIBETAN METHOD ... 62

23 REIKI LEVEL III ATTUNEMENT USUI/TIBETAN METHOD ... 63

Usui Tibetan Reiki Healing Energy Master / Teacher Student Manual

24	REIKI MASTER/TEACHER ATTUNEMENT USUI/TIBETAN METHOD	63
24.1	Key to abbreviations for notes in the previous section	64
25	REIKI WAIVER FORM	66
26	CHAKRA CRYSTALS	68
26.1	Garnet Crystal—Root Chakra	68
26.2	Carnelian Crystal—Sacral Chakra	68
26.3	Citrine Crystal—Solar Plexus Chakra	69
26.4	Rose Quartz Crystal-Heart Chakra,	70
26.5	Aquamarine Crystal—Throat Chakra	71
26.6	Amethyst Crystal—Third Eye Chakra	71
26.7	Clear Quartz—Crown Chakra	72
27	WHAT IS THE CAUSE OF A BLOCKED CHAKRA?	74
28	HOW DO I MAINTAIN CLEAR AND BALANCED CHAKRAS?	75
29	COURSE DESCRIPTIONS AND COSTS	78
29.1	How will being a Reiki practitioner benefit me?	78
29.2	Reiki Level I	78
29.3	Reiki Level II	79
29.4	Reiki Level III	80
29.5	Usui Tibetan Reiki Master/Teacher	81
30	CANADIAN REIKI ASSOCIATION	83
30.1	Common Voice	83
30.2	Affiliation	83
30.3	Certificate	83
30.4	Canadian Reiki Association Website Listing	83
30.5	Low-Cost Professional Liability Insurance	83
30.6	Discounts	84
30.7	Social Media and Newsletters	84
30.8	Student Members	84
30.9	Criteria for Registered Members	85
30.9.1	Registered Practitioners	85
30.9.2	Registered Teachers	85
30.10	Referrals for RP/RT-CRA	86
31	LISTINGS FOR RP/RT-CRA AT THE CANADIAN REIKI ASSOCIATION INTERNET PAGE	87

32 I BELIEVE………..88

1 Table of Tables

Table 1 Key to Abbreviations for Reiki Symbols 65

Usui Tibetan Reiki Healing Energy Master / Teacher Student Manual

Dr. Usui's Concepts and five Principles

1.1 Kanji

A system of Japanese writing using Chinese characters

招福の秘法,
萬病の霊薬.

今日丈けは:

    怒るな,

    心配すな,

    感謝して,

    業をはけめ,

    人に親切に.

        朝夕合掌して心に念じ,
        口に唱へよ.

        心身改善.
        臼井霊氣療法.

        肇祖,
        臼井甕男.

1.2 English

The secret art of inviting happiness,
The miraculous medicine for all diseases.

At least for today:

    Do not be angry,

    Do not worry,

    Be grateful,

    Work with diligence,

    Be kind to people.

        Every morning and evening, join your hands in meditation and pray with your heart.
        State in your mind and chant with your mouth.

        For improvement of mind and body.
        Usui Reiki Ryōhō.

The founder,
Mikao Usui.

2 Suggestions for Teaching

- Eat lightly or fast on the day of class. The emptier your body is, the more energy you can hold to pass attunements.

- Prepare yourself for passing attunement by increasing your energy—microcosmic orbit, meditation, and meditating on Antakarana.

- Attunement room—has crystals, candles, music, Tibetan bells, and incense if you wish—the more senses you engage in the initiate the richer the experience.

- Empty bladder before attunement process if contracting Hui Yin point.

- Make sure the attunement room is quiet—telephones turned off, etc.

- If sealing preparatory process before class, keeps everyone out of the room until attunement ceremony

- Clear glass for Water Ceremony using Sei He Ki and Chokurey

- Have students meditate before attunement—prepare them by quieting their minds

- The breath, the Hui Yin, tongue placement, and the Hara are all key points to do and hold automatically throughout all the attunements.

3 Reiki Master Mantra

The Reiki Master Mantra is said to be an empowerment which rings equal status with Usui or to bring forth Usui and all he stands for.

The mantra is:

> OM USUI SAMA HUNG

Rough translation:

Om = is associated with the energy of what can be seen

USUI = The guru or teacher

SAMA = equal or could also be a shortened version of a word like Samadhi, which is the space of pure consciousness

HUNG = is associated with heart/mind

It can be used anytime—during attunements, hands-on or absentee treatments to call forth greater energy; or, any other time to align with the fullness of the Reiki Mastership.

4 Michael's Sword Technique

The Michael Sword Technique is for healing emotional issues.

The first step is any healing, etheric, emotional/mental, spiritual, or physical is the client's verbal acknowledgement of imbalance or attachment, as this is an act of responsibility; a claiming of power. An attachment is actually an issue that has been created in the body, mind/energy complex and has not been successfully dealt with or eliminated at the causal level. Left on its own, the human body is more than capable of rebuilding itself continuously. It is only when a person habitually holds on to a pattern of imbalance, consciously or unconsciously, for the value that it derives, that disease becomes apparent. True healing begins with recognition and acceptance, and the client taking responsibility for his/her healing process.

The Michael Sword Technique uses and aligns the Reiki energy to help release, transmute, and uncover hidden memories related to a certain condition. This process is always successful whether the condition begins in this lifetime or another, and whether the client has a conscious recollection of when the issue started or not.

At the root of all issues/conditions are a series of disassociated memories. Healing cannot take place completely until the client can connect or associate all levels of these memories. Psychologists know that in order to change a habit, one must make it completely conscious.

Memories can take one of three forms disassociated, associated, or neuromuscular/tissue:

4.1 Disassociated memory

This may be subconscious or conscious and is usually the result of repression; situations and memories that are simply forgotten traumatic childhood issues, for instance. Left unattended and ignored for a time can create large energy blocks that eventually create disease and can lead to an untimely death, if not attended to.

4.2 Associated conscious memory

This is usually in the client's mind, and known to be connected with the issue/condition directly, but has not been dealt with directly.

4.3 Tissue or neuromuscular memory

This is the memory of events which are stored in the cells of tissue, particularly in muscle tissue. It has been found in research that the body can move because the muscles remember complex motion/action, and actually store and process hundreds of times more data than the brain. Most educational systems have discovered that if you can make learning practical and physical, the retention of new skills is substantially higher.

When the human body stores trauma, the area's self-healing abilities are diminished; the more trauma stored, the lower the flexibility and the longer for healing to occur. Once the different disassociated memories are revealed, connected, and released, then it is a simple matter for the body to make changes and create vibrant health once more. Reiki can perpetuate the changes; re-patterning emotional and mental programming on all levels. When the distant symbol is used in the energy re-patterning process, it works across time and space on the original cause, erasing it from the body's cellular memory.

Before beginning the session, discuss with the client that this technique used Reiki energy to reprogram the issue/condition in mind. It is unnecessary for the practitioner to know what the issue is, giving the client the space to accomplish the healing in the way s/he feels appropriate.

The wording of the phrases and questions is important, leading the client to retrieve the answers from deep within the psyche. Some well-formed questions to draw out inner answers are:

- "Why do I have this _____ issue?"
- "What is preventing the healing of _____?"
- "What is preventing me from feeling joy / peace, / intimacy in my life?"
- etc.

Any type of issue can be investigated and healed with the use of properly phrased questions. Inform the client to consider questions directly related to the healing of the issue; avoid questions that would/could trigger long, ongoing, and unsupportive answers, having little relation to the healing at hand.

The greatest boon this technique offers is its ability to assist the client in reaching a space that allows him/her to look objectively at their own issues in an environment free of pain, fear, and judgment. The technique does not force the client to face his/her fears and transgressions, but sets up the opportunity for the client to work on the issues subtly in their daily activities without reliving the trauma of the original experience.

5 Preparation

Begin by sharing the technique with the client and how it is performed; this helps lower the level of anticipation that the client may be experiencing. Then add a prayer of intent, empower yourself, the space, and the client. Treat the entire head, positions #1–4, and extra positions, if desired, to relax the client and start the energy flowing. Place your hands in the opening position

Usui Tibetan Reiki Healing Energy Master / Teacher Student Manual

OPENING HAND POSITION: left hand under the client's head, fingertips reach out of the skull, base of hand at the crown—right hand on top of the head, fingertips reaching over the forehead, base of hand at the crown.

Visually draw the Mental/Emotional Symbol, followed by the Power Symbol, on the back of your right hand. This accesses the client's subconscious mind and opens their energy field. It may leave them in a vulnerable state if the closing technique is not performed before ending the session. It is important to leave your left hand in its position during the entire technique and if you have to move, close the energy by spreading your fingers apart and lacing them on either side of the head

CLOSING HAND POSITION: base of hands together at the crown, fingertips reaching down each side of the head over each ear, all fingers lying flat except for the middle finger on both hands, which is bent and pointing into the head, balancing energy.

When the energy link between you and the client has been established, has the client visualizes a quiet scene in their mind, and projects their spirit to that place fully to experience it as if they were really there. Ask him/her to experience what their body would feel through the five senses if they were there. For the people not visually oriented, use a lot of sensory statements to activate their keenest sense. It is important that you know where the client's safe place of perfect peace is, so you can help to keep them there with occasional words and visual pictures. Have the client also create a screen or message board they can write on, and have them see or write in big, bold letters what the issue is that they have chosen to work on one issue per session.

When completed, has the client begins to scan their feet one leg at a time, creeping up the entire length of the leg; foot, ankle, calf, knee, and thigh. Memories are stored throughout the body, including the feet and legs, and may show themselves as sensations, feelings, colours, textures, or smells. Anything out of the ordinary maybe a repressed memory. As memories are discovered, have the client put them into a balloon, and have it float up above the body, still attached to the spot where the memory was discovered.

After both legs are completely done, have the client clear the central channel or spine by imagining a golden-white light entering the crown chakra and moving down the spine to the coccyx. As the light accumulates at the coccyx, it will begin to overflow out of the root chakra and have the client imagine the energy rising upward along a channel in front of the body. When it reaches the top of the body, have the client imagine the energy joining the Golden White light coming into the crown chakra, creating a continuous looping of the energy; cleansing, purifying, and opening the two main channels along the back and fronts of the body. Have the client realize the feelings and sensations being experienced.

Now have the client scan the rest of his/her body, ballooning any stored memories that are found. Guide the client through the entire body; the organs, hands, arms, shoulders, neck, and head. Once the client has identified and ballooned all appropriate memories discovered throughout the body, the next step is releasing the balloons, which represent cords or attachments to the memories. First, have the client will have to separate the soul from the physical body. Visualize or using their strongest sense imagine the spirit slipping out through the left side of their body. Then have them imagine floating to the left, above and a short distance from their body, observing it in a detached manner.

There are many methods that can be imagined cutting the attached balloons from the parts of the body where stored memories have been found; we are suggesting the use of the Flaming Blue Sword of Archangel Michael to accomplish the task. Ask the client to imagine reaching out with the left hand, receiving it from Michael, grasping it with both hands and gently swinging to sever the cords that hold the balloons. Begin at the feet and move up the entire body, remembering to also cut the balloons from the back. As each cord is cut, the client is to imagine the cord and the balloon bursting into violet flames, transmuting and burning away all traces of the memory inside the body. When the task is finished, have the client give the sword back to Archangel Michael, thanking him for his Flaming Blue Sword, which helped accomplish the complete detachment of all stored memories. Have the client converse with Michael, asking if there might be a message regarding the purification of the body from the attachments. Give ample time for this to happen.

Next, have the client imagine that his/her body is now filling up with golden-white light, beginning at the feet and moving upward to the crown. The light shines outward through the body, filling the auric field, disintegrating any leftover debris from the cord cutting. Next, have the spirit of the client approach the body and crawl to a horizontal position next to the physical body, and then slowly slip back into the body through the left side. Ask the client to focus on all parts of his/her body, paying close attention to any differences sensed or felt since the beginning of the exercise. Ask the client if the body feels lighter, with more freedom; ask about their emotional state of being.

Finish with the rest of the full-body treatment, asking the client to remain relaxed and in an open, loving state. The Reiki treatment will probably not take very long, as there is a lot of energy flowing through the meridians and chakras. Do the closing position,

CLOSING HAND POSITION: base of hands together at the crown, fingertips reaching down each side of the head over each ear, all fingers lying flat except for the middle finger on both hands, which is bent and pointing into the head, balancing energy

then cut the cords between you and the client's solar plexus and wash your hands/arms in cool water.

5.1 Helping the Client Understand

Spend a few minutes conversing with the client, supporting the choice to work on old issues, building his/her self-worth for following through with the technique. Explain the possible 3-2-1-day purification that will probably take place. The body has made changes on every level and will probably be in a state of shift and change for some time to come; the client needs to know that this could be uncomfortable, but no incapacitating. Ask the client to give you any feedback on the technique and particularly on how they are feeling.

Ask the client to monitor his/her emotions, physical reactions, and thoughts. If the conditions for which the client originally sought this technique continue to exist, then over one session may be needed to complete the process. Additional sessions can occur once a week for several weeks or several days in a row. It depends on the calendar availability of the client and the practitioner. It has been found, however, that stacking sessions within relatively short periods of time may actually begin simultaneous clearings, and can help to heal all levels of one's being in a more thorough, lasting manner.

6 Tree of Life Meditation

Begin by taking some full, deep breaths. Force nothing, just relax and breathe deeply. As you breathe, imagine yourself standing in a grove of tall trees within a deep forest. See yourself as one of those tall, sturdy trees. Breathe deeply and feel the ground beneath you and the sun shining down upon you. Feel your connection to the Earth and know you now have roots where your feet are.

Breathe deeply and on exhale, slowly begin to send those roots deep into the ground. Down, down through the grass and the topsoil, down through soil, rock, and the roots of other plants and trees, down through the many layers of Earth. Continue to send those roots down and down in search of the source at the centre of the Earth. Begin to feel the energy pulsating as you draw near and feel the heartbeat of the Earth.

When you reach that source of energy deep within the Earth, let it take a form in your mind's eye. It may be a huge crystal cluster, or the hot molten core of the Earth. With your roots, tap into that source of energy, breathe deeply and feel the energy slowly begin to rise, travelling up your roots. Up and up through the layers of Earth and soil and rock. Through roots, seedlings, and water tables. Feel the energy rise up through your roots, through your feet, your calves, and your thighs. Let that Mother Earth energy rise through your trunk, your torso, and up and up through your chest and arms and neck. Let it reach your head and simply fill you with her powerful energy. Stay with this feeling for a moment and just breathe.

Now, imagine you have branches that are tall and wide and reach up to the sky. Feel the air rushing around your branches and the warmth of the sun as it caresses your leaves. Take a deep breath and with it, take in the sky's energy and the sun. Let it touch and heal each leaf before being drawn into your branches. On another inhale, take that sky energy deep into your tree and feel it flow down through your head, your shoulders, your arms and chest. Breathe it into your torso, hips, and legs. Feel it mixing and mingling with the energies of the Earth. Stay with this feeling for a while and just breathe.

Feel yourself as being a conduit for Mother Earth energy together mixed with divine energy from Source. Feel the power of both energies within you become one together and one also with your energy—as all the energies of the universe unite within you, you become the energy of the universe. Ensure you continue to take your deep relaxing breaths in and also out for a few more minutes, allowing the energy to continue to surge through you.

When you are ready, slowly bringing your awareness back into the room, moving your head side to side, wiggling your fingers and moving your feet from side to side also and when you feel able to …. Opening your eyes feeling deeply relaxed and yet energized.

7 Chakras Invocation—First Time Invocation for Chakras

From the Light within and All that I Am from the Lord God of my Being and the bottom of my heart.

By the Divine Essence of my True Nature I now demand, in my name, and in the name of the Creator of all things.

That all Elements, all Emotions, all Memories and all Karma from any past life, and from this life, and from this day forward that are not conducive to my life mission, and in accord with my Higher Self now depart, go home, that you may serve others in your time as you have served me.

I release you with love, joy and gratitude for the service you have rendered me and the opportunity you have afforded me along my path of growth I now ask the Angels from the throne of Grace to take you back, where you belong.

In my name, and in the name of the Creator of all things, I now demand that my chakras be made open if they are closed, cleared if they are clogged, repaired if they are damaged, and brought into balance and harmony, centred and restored.

And that from this day forward they are the perfect receptors and transmitters and conductors to the limitless bounty of the Universe.

And that they bring to me only those things which are conducive to my life mission, in harmony with my desires and in full accord with my Higher Self, for this day on.

SO BE IT

Breathe deeply 3 cleansing breaths and say aloud
In with the Good, out with the Bad

Paul Carre,

Copyright waived

8   Second Time Invocation for Chakras

From the Light within and all that I Am from the Lord God of my Being and the bottom of my heart.

By the Divine Essence of my True Nature

I now demand, in my name, and in the name of the Creator of all things that all Elements, all Emotions, all Memories and all Karma from any past life, and from this life, and from this day forward that are not conducive to my life mission, and in accord with my Higher Self now depart, go home, that you may serve others in your time as you have served me.

I release you with love, joy and gratitude for the service you have rendered me and the opportunity you have afforded me along my path of growth I now ask the Angels from the throne of Grace to take you back, where you belong.

In my name, and in the name of the Creator of all things, I now demand that my chakras be made open if they are closed, cleared if they are clogged, repaired if they are damaged, and brought into balance and harmony, centred and restored.

And that from this day forward they are the perfect receptors and transmitters and conductors to the limitless bounty of the Universe.

And that they bring to me only those things which are conducive to my life mission, in harmony with my desires and in full accord with my Higher Self,
for this day on.

SO BE IT

Breathe deeply 3 cleansing breaths and say aloud
In with the Good, out with the Bad

Paul Carre,

Copyright waived

9 Grounding Meditation

- Sit with feet on the floor, back resting comfortably, focusing on tailbone

- Centre yourself. See yourself right to the core—the very essence of self that nothing can shake. Using your breath, breathing into the core and exhale, sending light through your body into every cell until all of you is filled with brilliant light.

- Place a dark coloured crystal between feet. This crystal provides an anchor for your energy and will keep you tied to the earth plane.

- Visualizing tree roots coming from under your feet—growing deep into the earth, travelling faster until they reach an enormous boulder—larger than any you have seen close to the centre of the Earth and anchor roots by winding them several times around the boulder.

- Drawing in a deep breath and feeling the heaviness and stability of that boulder's energy up through the tree roots. Feeling yourself deeply rooted to the Earth and being able to bring root energies up through your physical body, following your energy pathways, and expanding the energies around you and within you into the subtle body. Breathing in and drawing the energies through and around. Do this three times, take your time.

- You Will Feel Very Heavy and Very Grounded

- Visualize that the roots are released from the boulder. Bring your focus to heart centre

- Visualize a white ball of light from the centre of your chest radiating throughout your physical and subtle body. This light creates an energy balance for the grounding exercise.

- Bring awareness back into the room and clear the room of any energies that may have been released through the meditation

- drink plenty of water.

10 The Usui System of Attunements

This information is sacred. Do not show it to anyone or leave it where others could read it.

There are several differences between the original Usui system of attunements and the Usui/Tibetan system discussed previously in this manual. In the Usui/Tibetan System, the Tibetan symbols have been added along with the various healing techniques.

10.1 Reiki I—Initiatory Attunement

One of the major differences between the Reiki II attunements and I go into the hands.

In Reiki I, only the Power Symbol is put into the hands both when the hands are over the head and when they are open at the heart.

Before starting the actual attunement, have them sitting on a chair. You must be able to walk around the chair with legs uncrossed, fell flat on the floor, hands in prayer position at heart level, eyes closed. Explain that when tapped on the shoulder, they are to raise their hands to the top of the head. Standing in front of the initiate and say a silent prayer, invoking help from your spiritual guides, Reiki Masters and helpers, angels, light beings, etc. State to yourself and to them that this is to be the first attunement.

Draw the personal Mastery symbol on both your palms, say name 3 times, clap 3 times; then draw the power symbol on both palms, say name 3 times, and clap 3 times. Next draw the Power Symbol down the front of your body and over each of your chakras, saying a name 3 times for each open body to receive light. Draw all Reiki symbols into the air, fill, and seal the room with protective energy.

10.2 Attunement #1 of 4

10.2.1 Part One

1. Move behind; place both hands on top of the head, close your eyes, and meditate momentarily to gain rapport.

2. Draw the personal Mastery symbol over the crown, say name 3 times; guide the symbol with your dominant hand into their crown, the middle of the head, into the base of the brain. sweep

3. Touch the shoulder hands rise to crown

4. Draw the power symbol over the hands, repeat the name 3 times, and guide the symbol with your dominant hand into their hands, middle of the head and base of the brain sweep.

5. Gently nudge the hands forward to be returned to the heart

10.2.2 Part 2

1. Move to front, open the hands flat, holding them from beneath with your non-dominant hand. With your dominant hand, draw the Power Symbol in front of the third eye, say name 3 times, directing the symbol into the third eye 3 times. Pat

2. Draw the Power Symbol above the hands, direct the symbol into the hands 3 times, while saying the name 3 times. Then slap the hands lightly 3 times.

3. Bring the hands together and move them in front of the heart. Hold your hands over the hands and blow through them down to the solar plexus, up to the crown, back down to the solar plexus, and up to the hands one breath, one movement

4. moves to the next and repeats or go to part three.

10.2.3 Part 3

1. Move behind, place your hands-on shoulders, looking down through the crown chakra to the heart. Imagine a pink ball of light there and place a positive affirmation in the heart to be accepted by the start's subconscious mind; i.e. "You are a successful and empowered Reiki I practitioner, guided by divine love and wisdom." Repeat affirmation 3 times.

2. Bring your thumbs together, place them at the base of the start's skull, with fingers resting lightly on the neck. Visualize a door containing the Power Symbol being closed, say closing phrase 3 times; i.e. "I now seal this process with divine love and wisdom" Intend and feel the attunement completed, and the initiate connected to the Reiki source. Place your hands on the initiate's shoulders, feeling you both are blessed by the experience.

3. Move to the front, separate initiate's hands and place them on their heart. Move backwards three steps, put your hands into prayer position at your heart. Thank your guides and helpers. You may add a blessing for the initiate if you wish. Ask the initiate to take a deep breath and to slowly open their eyes. On eye contact, bow to them.

10.3 Attunement #2 of 4

The beginning procedure is the same unless stating the intent of which attunement you are about to perform. Tell your guides that this is Attunement II of the Reiki I Initiatory Attunements.

1. Move behind the initiate; place both hands on top of the head, close your eyes, and meditate momentarily to gain rapport.

2. Draw the personal Mastery symbol over the crown, say name 3 times; guide the symbol with your dominant hand into their crown, the middle of the head, into the base of the brain. sweep

3. Draw the distance symbol over the crown, say name 3 times, guide the symbols with your dominant hand into their crown, the middle of the head, into the base of the brain. Sweep.

4. Touch the initiate's shoulder hands rise to crown

5. Draw the power symbol over the hands, repeat the name 3 times, and guide the symbol with your dominant hand into their hands, middle of the head and base of the brain sweep.

6. Gently nudge the initiates hands forward to be returned to the heart

10.3.1 Part 2

1. Move to front, open the initiate's hands flat, holding them beneath with your non-dominant hand. With your dominant hand, draw the distance symbol in front of the third eye, say name 3 times, directing the symbol into the third eye 3 times. Repeat with power symbol.

2. Draw the Power Symbol above the hands, direct the symbol into the hands 3 times, while saying the name 3 times. Then slap the hands lightly 3 times.

3. Bring the initiate's hands together and move them in front of the heart. Hold your hands over the initiate's hands and blow through them down to the solar plexus, up to the crown, back down to the solar plexus, and up to the hands one breath, one movement.

10.4 Part 3

1. Move behind initiate, place your hands-on initiate's shoulders, looking down through the crown chakra to the heart. Imagine a pink ball of light there and place a positive affirmation in the

heart to be accepted by the initiate's subconscious mind; i.e. "You are a successful and empowered Reiki I practitioner, guided by divine love and wisdom." Repeat affirmation 3 times.

2. Bring your thumbs together, place them at the base of the initiate's skull, with fingers resting lightly on the neck. Visualize a door containing the Power Symbol being closed, say closing phrase 3 times; i.e. "I now seal this process with divine love and wisdom" Intend and feel the attunement completed, and the initiate connected to the Reiki source. Place your hands on the initiate's shoulders, feeling you both are blessed by the experience.

3. Move to the front, separate initiate's hands and place them on their heart. Move backwards 3 steps and put your hands into prayer position at your heart. Thank your guides and helpers. You may add a blessing for the initiate if you wish. Ask the initiate to take a deep breath and to slowly open their eyes. Upon eye contact, bow to them.

10.5 Attunement #3 of 4

The beginning procedure is the same unless stating the intent of which attunement you are about to perform. Tell your guides that this is Attunement III of the Reiki I Initiatory Attunements.

10.5.1 Part One

1. Move behind the initiate; place both hands on top of the head, close your eyes, and meditate momentarily to gain rapport.

2. Draw the personal Mastery symbol over the crown, say name 3 times; guide the symbol with your dominant hand into their crown, the middle of the head, into the base of the brain. sweep

3. Draw the mental/emotional symbol over the crown, say name 3 times, guide the symbols with your dominant hand into their crown, the middle of the head, into the base of the brain. Sweep.

4. Touch the initiate's shoulder hands rise to crown

5. Draw the power symbol over the hands, repeat the name 3 times, and guide the symbol with your dominant hand into their hands, middle of the head and base of the brain sweep.

6. Gently nudge the initiates hands forward to be returned to the heart

10.5.2 Part 2

1. Move to front, open the initiate's hands flat, holding them beneath with your non-dominant hand. With your dominant hand, draw the mental/emotional symbol in front of the third eye, say name 3 times, directing the symbol into the third eye 3 times. Repeat with power symbol.

2. Draw the Power Symbol above the hands, direct the symbol into the hands 3 times, while saying the name 3 times. Then slap the hands lightly 3 times.

3. Bring the initiate's hands together and move them in front of the heart. Hold your hands over the initiate's hands and blow through them down to the solar plexus, up to the crown, back down to the solar plexus, and up to the hands one breath, one movement

10.5.3 part three.

1. Move behind initiate, place your hands-on initiate's shoulders looking down through the crown chakra to the heart. Imagine a pink ball of light there and place a positive affirmation in the heart to be accepted by the initiate's subconscious mind; i.e. "You are a successful and empowered Reiki I practitioner, guided by divine love and wisdom," Repeat affirmation 3 times.

2. Bring your thumbs together, place them at the base of the initiate's skull, with fingers resting lightly on the neck. Visualize a door containing the Power Symbol being closed, say closing phrase 3 times; i.e. "I now seal this process with divine love and wisdom" Intend and feel the attunement completed, and the initiate connected to the Reiki source. Place your hands on the initiate's shoulders, feeling you both are blessed by the experience.

3. Move to the front, separate initiate's hands and place them on their heart. Move backwards 3 steps and put your hands into prayer position at your heart. Thank your guides and helpers. You may add a blessing for the initiate if you wish. Ask the initiate to take a deep breath and to slowly open their eyes. Upon eye contact, bow to them.

10.6 Attunement #4 of 4

The beginning procedure is the same unless stating the intent of which attunement you are about to perform. Tell your guides that this is Attunement III of the Reiki I Initiatory Attunements.

10.6.1 Part One

1. Move behind the initiate; place both hands on top of the head, close your eyes, and meditate momentarily to gain rapport.

2. Draw the personal Mastery symbol over the crown, say name 3 times; guide the symbol with your dominant hand into their crown, the middle of the head, into the base of the brain. Sweep

3. draw the distance symbol over the crown, say name 3 times, guide the symbols with your dominant hand into their crown, the middle of the head, into the base of the brain sweep. Repeat entire process with mental/emotional symbol

4. touch the initiate's shoulder hands rise to the crown.

5. Draw the power symbol over the hands, repeat the name 3 times, and guide the symbol with your dominant hand into their hands, middle of the head and base of the brain sweep.

6. Gently nudge the initiate's hand forward to be returned to the heart

10.6.2 Part 2

1. Move to front, open the initiate's hands flat, holding them beneath with your non-dominant hand. With your dominant hand, draw the distance symbol in front of the third eye, say name 3 times, directing the symbol into the third eye 3 times. Repeat with power symbol. Repeat entire process with mental/emotional symbol.

2. Draw the Power Symbol above the hands, direct the symbol into the hands 3 times, while saying the name 3 times. Then slap the hands lightly three times.

3. Bring the initiate's hands together and move them in front of the heart. Hold your hands over the initiate's hands and blow through them down to the solar plexus, up to the crown, back down to the solar plexus, and up to the hands one breath, one movement.

10.6.3 Part 3

1. Move behind initiate, place your hands-on initiate's shoulders, looking down through the crown chakra to the heart. Imagine a pink ball of light there and place a positive affirmation in the heart to be accepted by the initiate's subconscious mind; i.e. "You are a successful and empowered Reiki I practitioner, guided by divine love and wisdom." Repeat affirmation 3 times.

2. Bring your thumbs together, place them at the base of the initiate's skull, with fingers resting lightly on the neck. Visualize a door containing the Power Symbol being closed, say closing phrase 3 times; i.e. "I now seal this process with divine love and wisdom" Intend and feel the attunement completed, and the initiate connected to the Reiki source. Place your hands on the initiate's shoulders, feeling you both are blessed by the experience.

3. Move to the front, separate initiate's hands and place them on their heart. Move backwards 3 steps and put your hands into prayer position at your heart. Thank your guides and helpers. You may add a blessing for the initiate if you wish. Ask the initiate to take a deep breath and to slowly open their eyes. Upon eye contact, bow to them.

11 Reiki II—Initiatory Attunement

One difference between the Reiki I & II attunements goes into the hands.

In Reiki II, you will place three symbols into the hands both when the hands are over the head and open at the heart.

Before starting the actual attunement, have the initiate sitting on a chair. You must be able to walk around the chair with legs uncrossed, fell flat on the floor, hands in prayer position at heart level, eyes closed. Explain that when tapped on the shoulder, they are to raise their hands to the top of the head. Standing in front of the initiates, say a silent prayer, invoking help from your spiritual guides, Reiki Masters and helpers, angels, light beings, etc. State to yourself and to them that this is to be a Reiki Level II attunement.

Draw the personal Mastery symbol on both your palms, say the name 3 times, clap 3 times; then draw the power symbol on both palms, say name 3 times, and clap 3 times. Next draw the Power Symbol down the front of your body and over each of your chakras, saying the name 3 times for each open body to receive light. Drawing all Reiki symbols into the air fills and seals the room with protective energy

11.1 Part One.

1. Move behind the person; place both hands on top of the head, close your eyes, and meditate momentarily to gain rapport.

2. Draw the personal mastery symbol over the crown, say the name 3 times, and guide the symbol with your dominant hand into their crown, middle of the head and base of the brain.

3. Touch the initiate's shoulder hands raise to crown

4. Draw the distance symbol over the hands. Move the symbol with your dominant hand into their hands, crown and base of the brain sweep say the name 3 times. Repeat with Mental/Emotional Symbol and then Power Symbol.

5. Gently nudge the initiate's hands forward to be returned to the heart.

6. Move to the next initiate and repeat above, or do part two in only one initiate.

11.1.1 Part 2

1. Move to front, open the initiate's hands flat, holding them from beneath with your non-dominant hand. With your dominant hand, draw the distance symbol in front of forehead, say the name 3 times, directing symbol with your dominant hand into the third eye 3 times. Repeat with the Mental/Emotional and Power Symbols.

2. Draw the distance symbol above the hands, say the name 3 times, with your dominant hand guide the symbol into the hands 3 times, slap 3 times. Repeat with mental/emotional symbol and then with power symbol.

3. Bring the initiate's hands together and move them in front of the heart. Hold your hands over the initiate's hands and blow through them down to the solar plexus, up to the down, back down to the solar plexus and back to the hands. One breath, one movement

4. moves to the next initiate and repeats or goes to part three.

11.1.2 Part 3

1. Move behind the initiate, place your hands-on initiate's shoulders looking down through the crown chakra to the heart. Imagine a pink ball of light there and place a positive affirmation in the heart to be accepted by the initiate's subconscious mind; i.e. "You are a successful and confident Reiki Healer, guided by Divine Love and wisdom." Repeat affirmation 3 times.

2. Bring your thumbs together, place them at the base of the initiate's skull, with fingers resting lightly on the neck. Visualize a door containing the Power Symbol being closed, say a closing phrase, i.e. "I now seal this process with divine love and wisdom," repeat three times. Intend and feel the attunement completed, and the initiate connected to the Reiki source. Place your hands on the initiate's shoulders feeling you both are blessed by the experience.

3. Move to the front, separate the initiate's hands and place them on their heart

4. Move backwards three steps, put your hands into prayer position at your heart. Thank your guides and helpers. You can add a special blessing for the initiate. Ask the initiate to take a deep breath and to slowly open his/her eyes. Upon eye contact, bow to the newly initiated Reiki II practitioner.

11.2 Reiki III—Master/Teacher Initiatory Attunement

The difference between the Reiki I & II, and the Master/Teacher attunements goes into the hands and third eye. In Master/Teacher, the Personal Mastery Symbol and the other three symbols are placed into the hands both when the hands are over the head, and open at the heart and third eye.

Before starting the actual attunement, have the initiate sitting on a chair you must be able to walk around the chair with legs uncrossed, fell flat on the floor, hands in prayer position at heart level, eyes closed. Explain that when tapped on the shoulder, they are to raise their hands to the top of the head. Standing in front of the initiate, say a silent prayer, invoking help from your spiritual guides, Reiki Masters and helpers, angels, light beings, etc. State to yourself and to them that this is to be a Reiki Master/Teacher Initiatory Attunement.

Draw the personal Mastery symbol on both your palms, say the name 3 times, clap 3 times; then draw the power symbol on both palms, say name 3 times, and clap 3 times. Next draw the Power Symbol down the front of your body and over each of your chakras, saying names 3 times for each position open body to receive light. Drawing all Reiki symbols into the air fills and seals the room with protective healing energy

11.2.1 Part One.

1. Move behind the person, place both hands on top of the head, close your eyes, and meditate momentarily to gain rapport.

2. Touch the initiate's shoulder hands raise to crown

3. Draw the personal Mastery symbol over the hands, say name 3 times, and move the symbol with your dominant hand into their hands, the middle of the head and the base of the brain. Repeat with the Distant, Mental/Emotional, and Power Symbols.

4. Gently nudge the initiate's hands forward to be returned to the heart.

5. Move to the next person and repeat above, or do part two if only one initiate.

11.3 Part 2

1. Move to front, open the initiate's hands flat, holding them for beneath with your non-dominant hand. With your dominant hand, draw the Personal Mastery symbol in the air in front of the forehead, say name 3 times while directing the symbol with your hand into the third eye 3 times. Repeat with Distance, Mental/Emotional and Power Symbols.

2. Draw the Personal Mastery symbol over the hands, say name 3 times, direct the symbol into the hands 3 times, and slap 3 times. Repeat with the Distance, Mental/Emotional and Power Symbols.

3. Bring the initiate's hands together and move them back in front of the heart. Hold your hands over the initiate's hands and blow through them down to the solar plexus, up to the crown, down to the solar plexus and back to the hands. One breath, one movement

4. moves to the next initiate and repeats or goes to part three.

11.4 Part 3

1. Move behind initiate, place your hands-on initiate's shoulders, looking down through the crown chakra to the heart. Imagine a pink ball of light there and place a positive affirmation in the heart to be accepted by the initiate's subconscious mind. Repeat 3 times; i.e. "You are a successful and confident Reiki healer, guided by divine love and wisdom."

2. Bring your thumbs together, place them at the base of the initiate's skull with fingers resting lightly on the neck. Visualize a door containing the Power Symbol being closed, repeat a closing phrase 3 times; i.e. "I now seal this process with divine love and wisdom." Intend and feel the attunement completed, and the initiate connected to the Reiki source. Place your hands on the initiate's shoulders, feeling you both are blessed by the experience.

11.5 Part 4

1. Move to the front, separate initiate's hands and place on heart.

2. Move backwards 3 steps and put your hands into prayer position at your heart. Thank your guides and helpers. You can add a special blessing for the initiate. Ask the initiate to take a deep breath and slowly open their eyes. Upon eye contact, bow to the newly initiated Reiki Master.

12 Reiki Level I Initiatory Attunement Usui/Tibetan Method

One of the major differences between the Reiki II attunements and I go into the hands. In Reiki I for all 4 attunements only the power symbol is put into the hands both when the hands are over the head and when they are open at the heart.

Usui Tibetan Reiki Healing Energy Master / Teacher Student Manual

12.1 Attunement #1 of 4

1. Preparing yourself and the room for the Attunement Process

2. Say a silent prayer, invoking help from your spiritual guides, Reiki Masters, and helpers, light beings, angels, etc.

3. State to yourself and then that this is the first attunement of four Reiki I initiatory attunements.

4. Draw the personal mastery symbol on both palms, says the name three times, and clap three times.

5. Draw the power symbol on both palms, say name three times, and clap three times.

6. Draw the Power symbol down the front of the body and over each of your chakras saying name 3 times for each open body to receive light.

7. Drawing all six Reiki symbols into the air fills and seals the room with protective energy.

12.1.1 Preparing the Student for Attunement

1. Have students sit on a chair, you must be able to walk around the chair with legs uncrossed, feet flat on the floor, hands in prayer position at heart-level heart chakra, eyes closed.

2. Explain that when you tap on their shoulders, they are to raise their hands to the top of the head Crown Chakra.

3. Explain that when attunement is completed, you will bow to each other Namasté — 'The Divine in me greet and honours the Divine in you'.

12.1.2 Part One

1. Stand behind the student

2. With dominant hand make the sign of the fire serpent from the top of the head to the base of the spine; non-dominant hand holds energy at the side of the head.

3. Place both hands on the top of the student's head; close your eyes; meditate momentarily to gain rapport.

4. Do "Violet Breath"—put the tongue on the roof of the mouth, contract the Hui Yin point and continue to hold through the entire attunement; open your hands; exhales into the Crown Chakra, visualizing the Tibetan Master Symbol moving from the middle of your head, out with the breath and into the student's Crown Chakra; Repeat the name of the symbol 3 times while guiding the symbol with the dominant hand from the crown, through the middle of the head and into the base of the brain.

5. Draw the Personal Mastery Symbol over the Crown Chakra; say name 3 times, guide the symbol with the dominant hand into their Crown Chakra, middle of head and base of brain sweep.

6. Touch student's shoulder they raise their hands to Crown Chakra

7. Draw the Power symbol over the student's hands; say name 3 times, guide the symbol with dominant hand into their hands, middle of the head and base of the brain

8. Gently nudge the student's hands forward to Heart Chakra

12.1.3 Part 2—Stand in front of Student

1. Open the student's hands flat, holding them from beneath with your non-dominant hand; with dominant hand, draw the Power Symbol in front of third eye; say name 3 times, directing the symbol into the third eye 3 times.

2. Draw the Power Symbol above the hands; direct the symbol into the hands 3 times while saying the name 3 times; slap hands three times.

3. Bring students' hands together and move them back in front of the Heart Chakra; hold your hands over the student's hands; blow through the hands down to the solar plexus, up to the Crown Chakra, back down to the solar plexus and up to the hands one breath, one movement

12.1.4 Part Three—Stand behind Student

1. Place your hands-on student's shoulders looking down through crown chakra to the base of the spine.

2. Imagine a red ball of fire there and place a positive affirmation in the student's subconscious mind; "You are a successful and empowered Reiki I practitioner guided by Divine Love and Wisdom." Repeat affirmation 3 times.

3. Bring thumbs together and placed them at the back of the student's skull with fingers resting lightly on the neck. Visualize a door containing the Power symbol being closed and say the closing phrase 3 times: "I now seal this process with Divine Love and Wisdom." Intend and feel the attunement completed and the student connected to the Reiki source. Place your hands on the student's shoulders, feeling you are both blessed by the experience.

12.1.5 Part 4 — Stand in Front of the Student

1. Move to the front of the student. Hold your hands at waist level, palms facing students, inhale, and hold briefly, exhale releasing the Hui Yin and tongue. Intend the releasing energy to be a blessing for the student.

2. Move backwards three steps, put your hands into prayer position at your heart. Thank your guides and helpers. Ask the student to take a deep breath and to slowly open their eyes. Upon eye contact bow to them.

12.2 Attunement #2 of 4

1. Preparing yourself and the room for the Attunement process

2. Say a silent prayer, invoking help from your spiritual guides, Reiki Masters, and helpers, light beings, angels, etc.

3. State to yourself and then that this is the second attunement of four Reiki I initiatory attunements.

4. Draw the personal mastery symbol on both palms say the name 3 times. Clap 3 times

5. Draw the power symbol on both palms, say name three times, clap three times

6. Draw the Power symbol down the front of the body and over each of your chakras, saying name three times for each open body to receive light.

7. Draw all Reiki symbols into the air, fill, and seal the room with protective energy.

12.2.1 Preparing the Student for the Attunement

Usui Tibetan Reiki Healing Energy Master / Teacher Student Manual

1. Have students sit on a chair. You must be able to walk around the chair with legs uncrossed, feet flat on the floor, hands in prayer position at heart-level heart chakra, eyes closed.

2. Explain that when you tap on their shoulders, they are to raise their hands to the top of the head. Crown Chakra

3. Explain that when attunement is completed, you will bow to each other Namasté— "The Divine in me greets and honours the Divine in you."

Part One

1. With a dominant hand, make the sign of the fire serpent from the top of the head to the base of the spine; A non-dominant hand holds energy at the side of the head.

2. Place both hands on the top of the student's head, close your eyes, and mediate momentarily to gain rapport.

3. Do "Violet Breath"—Put tongue on the roof of the mouth, contract the Hui Yin point and continue to hold throughout the entire attunement. Open your hands, exhale into the Crown Chakra, visualizing the Tibetan Master Symbol moving from the middle of your head, out with the breath and into the student's Crown Chakra. Repeat the name of the symbol 3 times while guiding the symbol with the dominant hand from the crown, through the middle of the head and into the base of the brain.

4. Draw Personal Mastery Symbol over the Crown Chakra; Say name 3 times, guide the symbol with the dominant hand into their crown chakra, middle of the head and base of the brain.

5. Draw the Distance Symbol over the Crown Chakra. Say name 3 times, guide the symbol with the dominant hand into their crown Chakra, middle of the head and base of the brain.

6. Touch student's shoulder; they raise their hands to Crown Chakra.

7. Draw the power symbol over the students' hands, say name 3 times, and guide the symbol with dominant hand into their hands, middle of the head and base of the brain.

8. Gently nudge the students' hands forward to Heart Chakra

12.2.2 Part 2—Stand in front of Student

1. Open the student's hands flat, holding them from beneath with your non-dominant hand. With dominant hand, draw the distance symbol in front of the Third Eye; say name 3 times, directing

the symbol into the Third Eye three times. With dominant hand, draw the Power Symbol in front of the Third Eye. Say name 3 times, directing the symbol into the Third Eye 3 times.

2. Draw the power symbol above the hands. Direct the symbol into the hands 3 times while saying the name 3 times, slap 3 times

3. bring students' hands together and move them back in front of the heart chakra. Hold your hands over the student's hands. Blow through the hands down the solar plexus, up to the Crown Chakra, back down to the solar plexus and up to the hands one breath, one movement.

12.2.3 Part Three—Stand Behind the Student

1. Place your hands-on student's shoulders looking down through crown chakra to the base of the spine. Imagine a red ball of fire there and place positive affirmation in the student's subconscious mind; "You are a successful and empowered Reiki I practitioner guided by Divine Love and Wisdom." Repeat affirmation 3 times.

2. Bring thumbs together, place them at the back of the student's skull with fingers resting lightly on the neck; Visualize a door containing the Power symbol being closed. Say the closing phrase 3 times: "I now seal this process with Divine Love and Wisdom." Intend and feel the attunement completed and the student connected to the Reiki source. Place your hands on the student's shoulders, feeling you are both blessed by the experience.

12.2.4 Part 4—Stand in Front of Students

1. Move to the front of the student. Hold your hands at waist level, palms facing the student, inhale, and hold briefly, exhale, releasing the Hui Yin and tongue. Intend the releasing energy to be a blessing for the student.

2. Move backwards 3 steps and put your hands into prayer position at your heart. Thank your guides and helpers. Ask the student to take a deep breath and to slowly open their eyes. Upon eye contact, bow to them.

12.3 Attunement 3 of 4

1. Preparing yourself and the room for the Attunement process

2. Say a silent prayer, invoking help from your spiritual guides, Reiki Masters, and helpers, light beings, angels, etc.

3. State to yourself and then that this is the third attunement of four Reiki I initiatory attunements.

4. Draw the personal mastery symbol on both palms, says the name three times, and clap three times.

5. Draw the power symbol on both palms, say name three times, and clap three times.

6. Draw the Power symbol down the front of the body and over each of your chakras, saying name 3 times for each open body to receive light.

7. Draw all six Reiki symbols into the air, fill and seals the room with protective energy.

12.3.1 Preparing the Student for Attunement

1. Have students sit on a chair. You must be able to walk around the chair with legs uncrossed, feet flat on the floor, hands in prayer position at heart-level heart chakra, eyes closed.

2. Explain that when you tap on their shoulders, they are to raise their hands to the top of the head. Crown Chakra

3. Explain that when attunement is completed, you will bow to each other Namasté—'The Divine in me greet and honours the Divine in you."

12.3.2 Part One—Stand behind Student

1. With a dominant hand, make the sign of the fire serpent from the top of the head to the base of the spine; non-dominant hand holds energy at the side of the head.

2. Place both hands on the top of the student's head. Close your eyes and meditate momentarily to gain rapport.

3. Do "Violet Breath." Put tongue on the roof of the mouth, contract the Hui Yin point and continue to hold throughout the entire attunement. Open your hands, exhale into the Crown Chakra, visualizing the Tibetan Master Symbol Dumo moving from the middle of your head, out with the breath and into the student's Crown Chakra. Repeat the name of the symbol 3 times while guiding the symbol with the dominant hand from the crown, through the middle of the head and into the base of the brain.

4. Draw personal mastery symbol Daikoomyo over the Crown Chakra. Say name 3 times, guide the symbol with the dominant hand into their Crown Chakra. Middle of the head and base of the brain.

5. Draw mental/emotional symbol over the Crown Chakra. Say name 3 times, guide the symbol with the dominant hand into their Crown Chakra. Middle of the head and base of the brain

6. touch student's shoulder; they raise their hands to Crown Chakra.

7. Draw the power symbol over the student's hands, say name 3 times, and guide the symbol with dominant hand into their hands, middle of the head and base of the brain.

8. Gently nudge the student's hands forward to Heart Chakra

12.3.3 Part 2—Stand in front of students

1. Open the student's hands flat, holding them from beneath with your non-dominant hand. With dominant hand, draw the mental/emotional symbol in front of the third eye. Say name 3 times, directing the symbol into the Third Eye three times. With dominant hand, draw the Power Symbol in front of Third Eye, say name three times, directing the symbol into the Third Eye 3 times.

2. Draw the power symbol above the hands; Direct the symbol into the hands three times while saying the name 3 times; slap hands three times.

3. Bring students' hands together and move them back in front of Heart Chakra. Hold your hands over the student's hands, blow through the hands down to the solar plexus, up to the Crown Chakra, back down to the solar plexus and up to the hands one breath, one movement.

12.3.4 Part Three—Stand Behind the Student

1. Place your hands-on student's shoulder looking down through crown chakra to the base of the spine—Imagine a red ball of fire there and place positive affirmation in the student's subconscious mind; "You are a successful and empowered Reiki I practitioner guided by Divine Love and Wisdom." Repeat affirmation 3 times.

2. Bring thumbs together, place them at the back of the student's skull with fingers resting lightly on the neck; visualize a door containing the Power symbol being closed. Say the closing phrase 3 times: "I now seal this process with divine love and wisdom." Intend and feel the

attunement completed and the student connected to the Reiki source. Place your hands on the student's shoulders, feeling you are both blessed by the experience.

12.3.5 Part 4—Stand in Front of the Student

1. Move to the front of the student; Hold your hands at waist level, palms facing the student, inhale, and hold briefly, exhale, releasing the Hui Yin and tongue. Intend the releasing energy to be a blessing for the student.

2. Move backwards three steps, put your hands into prayer position at your heart. Thank your guides and helpers. Ask the student to take a deep breath and to slowly open their eyes. Upon eye contact, bow to them.

12.4 Attunement 4 of 4

1. Preparing yourself and the room for the Attunement process

2. Say a silent prayer, invoking help from your spiritual guides, Reiki Masters, and helpers, light beings, angels, etc.

3. State to yourself and then that this is the fourth attunement of four Reiki I initiatory attunements.

4. Draw the personal mastery symbol on both palms, say the name three times, and clap three times.

5. Draw the power symbol on both palms, say name three times, and clap three times.

6. Draw the power symbol down the front of the body and over each of your chakras, saying name 3 times for each open body to receive light.

7. Draw all six Reiki symbols into the air, fill, and seal the room with protective energy.

12.4.1 Preparing the Student for Attunement

1. Have students sit on a chair. You must be able to walk around the chair with legs uncrossed, feet flat on the floor, hands in prayer position at heart-level heart chakra, eyes closed.

2. Explain that when you tap on their shoulders, they are to raise their hands to the top of the head. Crown Chakra

3. Explain that when attunement is completed, you will bow to each other Namasté—'The Divine in me greet and honours the Divine in you."

12.4.2 Part One—Stand behind Student

1. With a dominant hand, make the sign of the fire serpent from the top of the head to the base of the spine; non-dominant hand holds energy at the side of the head.

2. Place both hands on the top of the student's head. Close your eyes and meditate momentarily to gain rapport.

3. Do "Violet Breath." Put tongue on the roof of the mouth, contract the Hui Yin point and continue to hold throughout the entire attunement. Open your hands, exhale into the Crown Chakra, visualizing the Tibetan Master Symbol Dumo moving from the middle of your head, out with the breath and into the student's Crown Chakra. Repeat the name of the symbol 3 times while guiding the symbol with the dominant hand from the crown, through the middle of the head and into the base of the brain.

4. Draw personal mastery symbol Daikoomyo over the Crown Chakra. Say name 3 times. Guide the symbol with the dominant hand into their Crown Chakra. Middle of the head and base of the brain.

5. Draw the distance symbol over the Crown Chakra. Say name 3 times, guide the symbol with the dominant hand into their crown chakra, middle of the head and base of the brain.

    Draw mental/emotional symbol over the Crown Chakra, say name 3 times, and guide the symbol with the dominant hand into their Crown Chakra, middle of the head and base of the brain.

6. Touch students' shoulders, they raise their hands to Crown Chakra

7. Draw the power symbol over the student's hands, say name 3 times, and guide the symbol with dominant hand into their hands, middle of the head and base of the brain.

8. Gently nudge the student's hands forward to Heart Chakra

12.4.3 Part 2—Stand in front of students

1. Open the student's hands flat, holding them from beneath with your non-dominant hand. With dominant hand, draw the distance symbol in front of the Third Eye, say name 3 times, directing the symbol into the Third Eye 3 times. With the dominant hand, draw the mental/emotional symbol in front of the third eye. Say name 3 times, directing the symbol into the Third Eye three times. With dominant hand, draw the Power Symbol in front of Third Eye, say name three times, directing the symbol into the Third Eye 3 times.

2. Draw the power symbol above the hands; Direct the symbol into the hands three times while saying the name 3 times; slap hands three times.

3. Bring students' hands together and move them back in front of Heart Chakra. Hold your hands over the student's hands, blow through the hands down to the solar plexus, up to the Crown Chakra, back down to the solar plexus and up to the hands one breath, one movement.

12.4.4 Part Three—Stand Behind the Student

1. Place your hands-on student's shoulder looking down through crown chakra to the base of the spine—Imagine a red ball of fire there and place positive affirmation in the student's subconscious mind; "You are a successful and empowered Reiki I practitioner guided by Divine Love and Wisdom." Repeat affirmation 3 times.

2. Bring thumbs together, place them at the back of the student's skull with fingers resting lightly on the neck; visualize a door containing the Power symbol being closed. Say the closing phrase 3 times: "I now seal this process with divine love and wisdom." Intend and feel the attunement completed and the student connected to the Reiki source. Place your hands on the student's shoulders, feeling you are both blessed by the experience.

12.4.5 Part 4—Stand in Front of the Student

1. Move to the front of the student; Hold your hands at waist level, palms facing the student, inhale, and hold briefly, exhale, releasing the Hui Yin and tongue. Intend the releasing energy to be a blessing for the student.

2. Move backwards 3 steps and put your hands into prayer position at your heart. Thank your guides and helpers. Ask the student to take a deep breath and to slowly open their eyes. Upon eye contact, bow to them.

13 Reiki Level II Initiatory Attunement Usui/Tibetan Method

One of the major differences between the Reiki I and II, attunements go into the hands. In Reiki II you will place three symbols into the hands, both when the hand is over the head and when they are open at the heart.

13.1 Preparing yourself and the room for the attunement process.

1. Say a silent prayer, invoking help from your spiritual guides, Reiki Masters, and helpers, light beings, angels, etc.

2. State to yourself and then that this is the Reiki II Initiatory Attunement.

3. Draw the personal mastery symbol on both palms, say the name three times, and clap three times.

4. Draw the power symbol on both palms, say name three times, and clap three times.

5. Draw the power symbol down the front of the body and over each of your chakras, saying name 3 times for each open body to receive light.

6. Draw all six Reiki symbols into the air, fill, and seal the room with protective energy.

13.1.1 Preparing the Student for Attunement

1. Have students sit on a chair. You must be able to walk around the chair with legs uncrossed, feet flat on the floor, hands in prayer position at heart-level heart chakra, eyes closed.

2. Explain that when you tap on their shoulders, they are to raise their hands to the top of the head. Crown Chakra

3. Explain that when attunement is completed, you will bow to each other Namasté—'The Divine in me greet and honours the Divine in you."

13.1.2 Part One—Stand behind the Student

1. With a dominant hand, make the sign of the fire serpent from the top of the head to the base of the spine; non-dominant hand holds energy at the side of the head.

2. Place both hands on the top of the student's head, close your eyes, and meditate momentarily to gain rapport.

3. Do "Violet Breath." Put tongue on the roof of the mouth, contract the Hui Yin point and continue to hold throughout the entire attunement. Open your hands and exhale into the Crown Chakra, visualizing the Tibetan Master Symbol moving from the middle of your head, out with the breath and into the student's Crown Chakra. Repeat the name of the symbol 3 times while guiding the symbol with the dominant hand from the crown, through the middle of the head and into the base of the brain.

4. Draw Personal Mastery Symbol over the Crown Chakra; Say name 3 times, guide the symbol with the dominant hand into their crown Chakra, middle of the head and base of the brain.

5. Touch student's shoulder; they raise their hands to Crown Chakra.

6. Draw the distance symbol over the hands, say name 3 times, and guide the symbol with the dominant hand into their hands, middle of the head and base of the brain. Draw the mental/emotional symbol over the hands, say name 3 times, and guide the symbol with the dominant hand into their hands, middle of the head and base of the brain. Draw the power symbol over the student's hands, say name 3 times, and guide the symbol with the dominant hand into their hands, middle of the head and base of the brain.

7. Gently nudge the student's hands forward to Heart Chakra.

13.1.3 Part 2—Stand in front of Student

1. Open the student's hands flat, holding them from beneath with your non-dominant hand. With dominant hand, draw the distance symbol in front of the Third Eye; say name 3 times, directing the symbol into the Third Eye 3 times. With dominant hand, draw the mental/emotional symbol in front of the Third Eye, say name 3 times, directing the symbol into the Third Eye 3 times. With dominant hand, draw the Power Symbol in front of the Third Eye, say name 3 times, directing the symbol into the third eye 3 times.

2. Draw the distance symbol above the hands, direct the symbol into the hands 3 times while saying the name 3 times, and slap hands 3 times. Draw the mental/emotional symbol above the hands. Direct the symbol into the hands 3 times while saying the name 3 times, slap hands 3 times. Draw the Power symbol above the hands, direct the symbol into the hands 3 times while saying the name 3 times, and slap hands 3 times.

3. Bring students' hands together and move them back in front of the heart chakra. Hold your hands over the student's hands, blow through the hands down to the solar plexus chakra, up to the Crown chakra, back down to the solar plexus chakra and up to the hands one breath, one movement.

13.1.4 Part Three — Stand Behind the Student

1. Place your hands-on student's shoulders looking down through crown chakras to the base of the spine. Imagine a red ball of fire there and place positive affirmation in the student's subconscious mind: "You are a successful and empowered Reiki II practitioner guided by Divine Love and Wisdom." Repeat affirmation 3 times.

2. Bring thumbs together and place them at the back of the student's skull with fingers resting lightly on the neck. Visualize a door containing the Power Symbol being closed. Say the closing phrase 3 times, "I now seal this process with Divine Love and Wisdom." Intend and feel the attunement completed and the student connected to the Reiki source. Place your hands on the student's shoulders, feeling you are both blessed by the experience.

13.1.5 Part 4 — Stand in Front of the Student

1. Move to the front of the student; Hold your hands at waist level, palms facing the student, inhale, and hold briefly, exhale, releasing the Hui Yin and tongue. Intend the releasing energy to be a blessing for the student.

2. Move backwards 3 steps and put your hands into prayer position at your heart. Thank your guides and helpers. Ask the student to take a deep breath and to slowly open their eyes. Upon eye contact, bow to them.

Usui Tibetan Reiki Healing Energy Master / Teacher Student Manual

14 Reiki Level III Initiatory Attunement Usui/Tibetan Method

The difference between the Reiki I & II attunements and the III is what goes into the hands and third eye. In III, the Personal Mastery symbol and the other three symbols are placed into the hands both when the hands are over the head, and open at the heart and the third eye.

Before starting the actual attunement, have the initiate sitting on a chair. You must be able to walk around the chair, with legs uncrossed, feet flat on the floor, hands in prayer position at heart level, eyes closed. Explain that when tapped on the shoulder, they are to raise their hands to the top of the head. Standing in front of the initiates, say a silent prayer, invoking help from your spiritual guides, Reiki Masters and helpers, angels, light beings, etc. State to yourself and to them that this is to be a Reiki III Initiatory Attunement.

Draw the Personal Mastery Symbol on both your palms, say name 3 times, clap 3 times, then draw the Power Symbol on both palms, say name 3 times, clap 3 times. Next draw the Power Symbol down the front of your body, and over each of your chakras, saying names 3 times for each position opens the body to receive light. Drawing all six Reiki symbols into the air fills and seals the room with protective, healing energy.

14.1 Part One

1. Move behind the person; with the dominant hand, make the sign of the fire serpent, from the top of the head, down to the base of the spine, a non-dominant hand holds energy at the side of the head.

2. Place both hands on top of the head, close your eyes, and meditate momentarily to gain rapport.

3. Do the "Violet Breath." Put tongue on the roof of the mouth, contract the Hui Yin point, and continues to hold throughout the entire attunement. Open your hands and exhale into the Crown Chakra, visualizing the Tibetan Master Symbol moving from the middle of your head, out with the breath and into the student's Crown Chakra. Repeat the name of the symbol 3 times while guiding the symbol with the dominant hand from the crown. Through the middle of the head and into the base of the brain.

4. Touch students' shoulders; they raise their hands to Crown Chakra.

5. Draw the personal Mastery symbol over the hands, say name 3 times; move the symbol with your dominant hand into their hands, the middle of the head and the base of the brain. Repeat with the Distant, Mental/Emotional and Power Symbols.

6. Gently nudge the initiate's hands forward to be returned to the heart.

7. Move to the next person and repeat above or do part two, if only one initiate.

14.1.1 Part 2—Stand in front of Student

1. Open the student's hands flat, holding them from beneath with your non-dominant hand. With the dominant hand, draw the Personal Mastery Symbol in front of the Third Eye. Say the name 3 times while directing the symbol with your hand into the third eye 3 times. Distance symbol in front of the Third Eye; say name 3 times, directing the symbol into the Third Eye 3 times. With dominant hand, draw the mental/emotional symbol in front of the Third Eye, say name 3 times, directing the symbol into the Third Eye 3 times. With dominant hand, draw the Power Symbol in front of the Third Eye, say name 3 times, directing the symbol into the third eye 3 times.

2. Draw the Personal Mastery symbol over the hands, say name 3 times, direct the symbol into the hands 3 times, and slap 3 times. Draw the distance symbol above the hands, direct the symbol into the hands 3 times while saying the name 3 times, and slap hands 3 times. Draw the mental/emotional symbol above the hands. Direct the symbol into the hands 3 times while saying the name 3 times, slap hands 3 times. Draw the Power symbol above the hands, direct the symbol into the hands 3 times while saying the name 3 times, and slap hands 3 times.

3. Bring students' hands together and move them back in front of the heart chakra. Hold your hands over the student's hands, blow through the hands down to the solar plexus chakra, up to the Crown chakra, back down to the solar plexus chakra and up to the hands one breath, one movement.

14.1.2 Part Three—Stand Behind the Student

1. Place your hands-on student's shoulders looking down through crown chakras to the base of the spine. Imagine a red ball of fire there and place positive affirmation in the student's subconscious mind: "You are a successful and empowered Reiki III practitioner guided by Divine Love and Wisdom." Repeat affirmation 3 times.

2. Bring thumbs together and place them at the back of the student's skull with fingers resting lightly on the neck. Visualize a door containing the Power Symbol being closed. Say the closing phrase 3 times, "I now seal this process with Divine Love and Wisdom." Intend and feel the attunement completed and the student connected to the Reiki source. Place your hands on the student's shoulders, feeling you are both blessed by the experience.

14.1.3 Part 4—Stand in Front of the Student

1. Move to the front of the student; Hold your hands at waist level, palms facing the student, inhale, and hold briefly, exhale, releasing the Hui Yin and tongue. Intend the releasing energy to be a blessing for the student.

2. Move backwards 3 steps and put your hands into prayer position at your heart. Thank your guides and helpers. Ask the student to take a deep breath and to slowly open their eyes. Upon eye contact, bow to them.

15 Reiki Master/Teacher Attunement Usui/Tibetan Method

The difference between the Reiki I and II and the Master/Teacher attunements goes into the hands and the Third Eye. In Master/Teacher, the Personal Mastery Symbol and the other three symbols are placed into the hands both when the hands are over the head and open at the heart and the Third Eye.

15.1 Preparing yourself and the room for the Attunement process

1. Meditation and water ceremony optional—see notes after Attunement description
2. Say a silent prayer, invoking help from your spiritual guides, Reiki Masters, and helpers, light beings, angels, etc.
3. State to yourself and then that this is the Reiki Master/Teacher Initiatory Attunement.
4. Draw the personal mastery symbol on both palms, say the name three times, and clap three times.
5. Draw the power symbol on both palms, say name three times, and clap three times.
6. Draw the power symbol down the front of the body and over each of your chakras, saying name 3 times to receive light.
7. Draw all six Reiki symbols into the air, fill, and seal the room with protective energy.

15.1.1 Preparing the Student for Attunement

1. Have students sit on a chair. You must be able to walk around the chair with legs uncrossed, feet flat on the floor, hands in prayer position at heart-level heart chakra, eyes closed.
2. Explain that when you tap on their shoulders, they are to raise their hands to the top of the head. Crown Chakra
3. Explain that when attunement is completed, you will bow to each other Namasté—'The Divine in me greet and honours the Divine in you."

15.1.2 Part One

Usui Tibetan Reiki Healing Energy Master / Teacher Student Manual

1. With a dominant hand, make the sign of the fire serpent from the top of the head to the base of the spine. A non-dominant hand holds energy at the side of the head.

2. Place both hands on the top of the student's head, close your eyes, and meditate momentarily to gain rapport.

3. Touch students' shoulders, they raise their hands to Crown Chakra

4. Place your hands around student's hands—do "Violet Breath." Put tongue on the roof of the mouth, contract the Hui Yin point and continue to hold throughout the entire attunement, open your hands and exhale over the hands, visualizing the Tibetan Master Symbol, moving from the middle of your head, out with the breath and into the student's hands. Repeat the name of the symbol 3 times while guiding the symbol with the dominant hand from the hands, through the middle of the head and into the base of the brain.

5. Draw Fire serpent symbol over the hands, say name 3 times, and guide the symbol with the dominant hand into their hands, middle of the head and base of the brain.

    a. Repeat the process for each symbol individually Raku, Ran Sei and Ren So Mei.

    b. Repeat the process for each symbol individually Personal Mastery Symbol, Distance, Mental/Emotional and Power Symbol.

6. Gently nudge the student's hands forward to Heart Chakra.

15.1.3 Part 2—Stand in front of Student

1. Open the hands flat, holding them from beneath with your non-dominant hand. With dominant hand, draw the Tibetan Master Symbol in front of the Third Eye, say name 3 times, directing the symbol into the third eye 3 times.

    a) Repeat the process for each symbol individually Fire Serpent, Raku, Ran Sei, and Ren So Mei.

    b) Repeat the process for each symbol individually personal mastery, distance, mental/emotional and power symbol.

2. Draw the Tibetan Master Symbol above the hands, direct the symbol into the hands 3 times while saying the name 3 times, and slap hands 3 times.

a) Repeat the process for each symbol individually Fire Serpent, Raku, Ran Sei, and Ren So Mei.

b) Repeat the process for each symbol individually personal mastery, distance, mental/emotional and power symbol.

3. Bring students' hands together and move them back in front of the Heart Chakra. Hold your hands over the student's hands, blow through the hands down to the solar plexus, up to the Crown chakra, back down to the solar plexus and up to the hands one breath, one movement.

15.1.4 Part Three — Stand Behind the Student

1. Place your hands-on student's shoulders looking down through crown chakra to the base of the spine. Imagine a red ball of fire there and place positive affirmation in the student's subconscious mind. "You are a successful and confident Reiki Master/Teacher guided by divine love and wisdom." Repeat affirmation 3 times.

2. Bring thumbs together and place them at the back of the student's skull with fingers resting lightly on the neck. Visualize a door containing the power symbol being closed. Say the closing phrase 3 times: "I now seal this process with divine love and wisdom." Intend and feel the attunement completed and the student connected to the Reiki source. Place your hands on the student's shoulders, feeling you are both blessed by the experience.

15.1.5 Part 4 — Stand in Front of Students

1. Move backwards three steps. Put your hands in the prayer position at your Heart Chakra. Thank your guides and helpers.

2. Ask the student to take a deep breath and to slowly open their eyes. Upon eye contact, bow to the new Reiki Master/Teacher.

Usui Tibetan Reiki Healing Energy Master / Teacher Student Manual

16 Water Ceremony and Meditation—Master/Teacher Attunement

16.1 Optional Meditation for Master/Teacher Attunement

Doing this meditation before the attunement takes students into a deep meditative state and prepares them for the attunement process.

Getting comfortable and staring straight ahead of you with your eyes open … now close your eyes. Take a deep breath and as you exhale, relax your entire body. Feel your face relax. Feel your arms relax. Feel your legs relax. Feel your whole body relaxed.

As I count from 10 to 1, you will feel your entire body relaxing even more … 10 - 9 - 8—more and more relaxed 7 - 6-5- completely relaxed 4 - 3 - 2—deeper and deeper into relaxation - 1—you are now completely relaxed and ready to raise your vibrational rate … with feelings of love … and strong positive thoughts…. You may do this by surrounding yourself with a beautiful protective white light…. This white light is a vibrant white light…. See it entering your body now through your crown chakra and spreading all the way down your body to the base of your spine. Feel yourself surrounded and full of this beautiful, vibrant, white light. Now see this white light extending out of your body in all directions out into the universe and as you do, you experience you are one with the universe, one with ALL THAT IS.

Now, keep your eyes closed and bring your hands in the prayer position up the Heart Chakra as we begin the Reiki Master/Teacher Attunement process. Proceed with Attunement

16.2 Water Ceremony Optional for Reiki Master/Teacher Attunement

Have the student or students take part in the Water Ceremony, which symbolizes the rebirth of spirit into matter and enhances the flow of energy through the body. The water should be distilled or spring water mixed with juice from 1 to 2, a fresh lemon added for each 8 oz. Of water and should be served at room temperature. Master prepares water by doing Violet's breath and "blowing" the Master symbol into the water. This changes the vibration of the water. If possible, use a special glass that is only used for this ceremony so that the vibrations of the glass are specifically dedicated to the Water Ceremony. I regardless of whether you use a specific glass, clear the vibrations before every use by drawing SeiHeKi and Chokurey over the glass.

This ceremony cleanses students internally to prepare for attunement.

Pour a glass of water for each student. Instruct them to hold the glass between their hands at the solar plexus level.

Ask them to take a deep breath and hold it.

Instruct them to close their eyes, visualize the colour blue intensely, and exhale with force against the front teeth, which will make a hissing sound. During exhaling, they should visualize the blue as a mist passes from the breath into the water. During breathing, the Master places his/her left hand on the initiate's crown chakra and implants the SeiHeKi symbol into the subconscious mind by using the Violet Breath.

Have students hold the glass in their left hand and with the right make a Chokurey horizontally over the rim of the glass and repeat the name 3 times. Have them repeated aloud,

> "I invoke the Spirit of the Water to receive the Divine Benediction of Fire. That as I partake of this water, so shall I receive the Divine Benediction of Fire."

Then the student makes a Chokurey over the top of the glass vertically, repeats the name 3 times and drinks the water.

17 Usui Reiki Level I Teaching Notes

1. Opening/Introductions/Question period

2. Overview of schedule

3. History of Reiki

4. Reiki Principles

5. Chakras

6. Usui Reiki Level I Attunement

    Lunch Break

7. Review Reiki Self-treatment

8. Practise Self Reiki session—All

9. Review Healing Other Reiki sessions

10. Practice Healing Other sessions

11. Discuss Reiki Values for Success

12. Hand out certificates

13. Congratulations and welcome to Usui Shiki Ryoho!

18 Usui Reiki Level II Teaching Notes

1. Opening/Introductions/Question period
2. Outline schedule for day
3. Usui Reiki II Attunement
4. Introduction to Second Degree Reiki
5. Learning the Symbols
    - Trace/say symbols on page
    - Draw/say symbols on paper
    - Draw/say symbols in air
    - Draw/say symbols in mind's eye

    Break

6. Chakra Balancing Technique
7. Distance Healing Session

    Lunch

8. Marma points and Reiki
9. Healing Crystals and Reiki
10. Manifesting Goals—Creating prosperity with Reiki exercise
11. Storing energy for continuous treatments
12. Practice sessions using symbols
13. Congratulations! and hand out certificates

Usui Tibetan Reiki Healing Energy Master / Teacher Student Manual

19   Usui Reiki Level III Teaching Notes

- Usui Reiki Master Practitioner, Usui/Tibetan Advanced Reiki Training

1. Opening/Introductions/Question period
2. Reiki Level III Attunement
3. Reiki purification process
4. Personal Mastery Symbol
5. Dr. Usui's Healing Techniques
6. Usui/Tibetan Symbols
7. The Hara
8. The Hui Yin
9. The Violet Breath
10. Etheric Cleansing

   Lunch

11. Microcosmic Orbit
12. Meditation—Microcosmic Orbit
13. Reiki Healing Attunements
14. Practical time—Healing Attunement observes whole attunement by Master
15. Crystal Tower Grids
16. Antahkarana symbol
17. Questions
18. Congratulations! Hand out certificates

20 Usui/Tibetan Reiki Master/Teacher Teaching Notes

1. Opening/Introductions/Question period
2. Attunement Meditation
3. Water Ceremony
4. Reiki Master/Teacher Attunement

   Break

5. Dr. Usui's Concepts and five Principal
6. Suggestions for Teaching
7. Reiki Master Mantra

   Lunch

8. Meditations by Reiki Master/Teacher Students
9. Michael's Sword Technique
10. Tree of Life Meditation
11. Chakra Invocations
12. Presentations by Reiki Master/Teacher Students
13. Usui Attunements
14. Usui/Tibetan Attunements
15. Water ceremony & meditation
16. Teaching Notes
17. Attunement Guide
18. Practice session—Attunements
19. Congratulations! Hand out certificates
20. Question Period

21. Canadian Reiki Association

Usui Tibetan Reiki Healing Energy Master / Teacher Student Manual

21 Attunement Guide

21.1 REIKI LEVEL I ATTUNEMENT USUI/TIBETAN METHOD

1. prep room centre, DKM palms, CHO palms, CHO self, CHO chakras — draw 6 symbols H, S, C/D, FS, R

21.2 Attunement 1/4

1. behind
2. FS down the spine
3. both hands @ crown
4. VB, HY
5. open hands — exhale to crown blowing DUMO to students' crown — say/sweep 3x
6. draw DKM — say/sweep 3x
7. touch shoulders — hands to crown
8. draw CHO say/sweep 3x
9. nudge hands to heart

1. front
2. open hands
3. draw CHO over third eyes — say/pat 3x
4. draw CHO over hands — say/slap hands 3x
5. bring students' hands together
6. blow through hands — SP, CR blow through hands — SP, CR heart

1. behind
2. look through crown to base of spine — red ball of fire
3. "You are a successful and confident Reiki Level I guided by Divine love and wisdom" 3x
4. thumbs — CHO — door "I now seal this process with Divine love and wisdom" 3x
5. blessing

1. front
2. palms forward — release HY — blessing
3. moves back 3 steps — hands in prayer — open eyes — Namasté

21.3 Attunement 2/4

1. behind
2. FS down the spine
3. both hands @ crown

4. VB, HY
5. open hands—exhale to crown blowing DUMO to students' crown—say/sweep 3x
6. draw DKM over crown—say/sweep 3x
7. draw HON over crown—say/sweep 3x
8. touch shoulders—hands to crown
9. draw CHO say/sweep 3x
10. nudge hands to heart

1. front
2. open hands
3. draw HON over third eye—say/pat 3x
4. draw CHO over third eye—say/pat 3x
5. draw CHO over hands—say/slap hands 3x
6. bring students' hands together
7. blow through hands—SP, CR heart

1. behind
2. look through crown to base of spine—red ball of fire
3. "You are a successful and confident Reiki Level I guided by Divine Love and wisdom" 3x
4. thumbs—CHO—door "I now seal this process with Divine love and wisdom" 3x
5. blessing

1. front
2. palms forward—release HY—blessing
3. moves back 3 steps—hands in prayer—open eyes—Namasté

21.4 Attunement

1. behind
2. FS down the spine
3. both hands @ crown
4. VB, HY
5. open hands—exhale to crown blowing DUMO to students' crown—say/sweep 3x
6. draw DKM over crown—say/sweep 3x
7. draw SHK over crown—say/sweep 3x
8. touch shoulders—hands to crown
9. draw CHO say/sweep 3x
10. nudge hands to heart

1. front
2. open hands
3. draw SHK over third eye—say/pat 3x

4. draw CHO over third eye—say/pat 3x
5. draw CHO over hands—say/slap hands 3x
6. bring students' hands together
7. blow through hands—SP, CR, and heart

1. behind
2. look through crown to base of spine—red ball of fire
3. "You are a successful and confident Reiki Level I guided by Divine Love and wisdom" 3x
4. thumbs—CHO—door "I now seal this process with Divine love and wisdom" 3x
5. blessing

1. front
2. palms forward—release HY—blessing
3. moves back 3 steps—hands in prayer—open eyes—Namasté

21.5 Attunement 4/4

1. behind
2. FS down the spine
3. both hands @ crown
4. VB, HY
5. open hands—exhale to crown blowing DUMO to students' crown—say/sweep 3x
6. draw DKM over crown—say/sweep 3x
7. draw HON over crown—say/sweep 3x
8. draw SHK over crown—say/sweep 3x
9. touch shoulders—hands to crown
10. draw CHO say/sweep 3x
11. nudge hands to heart

1. front
2. open hands
3. draw HON over third eye—say/pat 3x
4. draw SHK over third eye—say/pat 3x
5. draw CHO over third eye—say/pat 3x
6. draw CHO over hands—say/slap hands 3x
7. bring students' hands together
8. blow through hands—SP, CR, SP, heart

1. behind
2. look through the crown to the base of the spine—a red ball of fire
3. looks through crown to heart chakra—pink ball of love and compassion
4. "You are a successful and confident Reiki Level I guided by Divine Love and wisdom" 3x

5. thumbs—CHO—door "I now seal this process with Divine love and wisdom" 3x
6. blessing

1. front
2. palms forward—release HY—blessing
3. moves back three steps—hands in prayer—open eyes—Namasté

22 Reiki Level Ii Attunement Usui/Tibetan Method

1. prep room centre, DKM palms,
2. CHO palms, CHO self, and CHO chakras—draw six symbols H, S, C/D, FS, R

1. behind
2. FS down the spine
3. both hands @ crown
4. VB, HY
5. open hands—exhale to crown blowing DUMO to students' crown—say/sweep 3x
6. draw DKM—say/sweep 3x
7. touch shoulders—hands to crown
8. draw HON say/sweep 3x
9. repeat for each SHK. CHO
10. nudges hands to heart

1. front
2. open hands
3. draw HON over third eye—say/pat 3x
4. repeat for each SHK, CHO
5. draws HON over hands—say/slap hands 3x
6. repeat for each SHK, CHO
7. brings students' hands together
8. blows through hands—SP, CR, SP, heart

1. behind
2. look through the crown to the base of the spine—a red ball of fire
3. looks through crown to heart chakra—pink ball of love and compassion
4. "You are a successful and confident Reiki Level II guided by Divine Love and wisdom" 3x
5. thumbs—CHO—door "I now seal this process with Divine love and wisdom" 3x
6. blessing

1. front
2. palms forward—release HY—blessing
3. moves back 3 steps—hands in prayer—open eyes—Namasté

Usui Tibetan Reiki Healing Energy Master / Teacher Student Manual

23 Reiki Level Iii Attunement Usui/Tibetan Method

1. prep room centre,
2. DKM palms,
3. CHO palms,
4. CHO self,
5. CHO chakras — draw 6 symbols H, S, C/D, FS, R

1. behind
2. FS down the spine
3. both hands @ crown
4. VB, HY
5. visualize DUMO to students' crown — say/sweep 3x
6. touch shoulders — hands to crown
7. draw FS to hands — say/sweep 3x
8. draw Ran Sai — say/sweep 3x
9. draw Ren So Mai — say/sweep 3x
10. draw DKM, say/sweep 3x
11. repeat for each HON, SHK, and CHO
12. nudge hands to heart

1. front
2. open hands
3. draw Dumo over third eye — say 3 x — pat 3x
4. repeat FS, Ran Sai, Ren So Mai, DKM, ON, SHK, CHO
5. draw Dumo over hands — say/slap hands 3x
6. repeat FS, Ran Sai, Ren So Mai, DKM, ON, SHK, CHO
7. brings students' hands together
8. blow through hands — SP, CR, SP, heart

1. behind
2. look through the crown to the base of the spine — a red ball of fire
3. looks through crown to heart chakra — pink ball of love and compassion
4. "You are a successful and confident Reiki Master Practitioner guided by Divine Love and wisdom" 3x
5. thumbs — CHO — door "I now seal this process with Divine love and wisdom" 3x
6. blessing

1. front
2. palms forward — release HY — blessing
3. moves back three steps — hands in prayer — open eyes — Namasté

24 Reiki Master/Teacher Attunement Usui/Tibetan Method

Usui Tibetan Reiki Healing Energy Master / Teacher Student Manual

1. Prep room centre,
2. DKM palms,
3. CHO palms,
4. CHO self,
5. CHO chakras—draw 6 symbols H, S, C/D, FS, R

1. behind
2. FS down the spine
3. both hands @ crown
4. touch shoulders—hands to crown
5. VB, HY
6. open hands, visualize DUMO to students' hands—say/sweep 3x
7. Draw DKM—say/sweep 3x
8. Draw Hon—say/sweep 3x
9. Draw SHK—say/sweep 3x
10. Draw CHO—say/sweep 3x
11. nudge hands to heart

1. front
2. open hands—
3. draw over third eye—say 3 x—pat 3x DKM, ON, SHK, CHO
4. draws over hands—say 3 x—pat 3x DKM, ON, SHK, CHO
5. brings students' hands together
6. blow thru hands—SP, CR, heart

1. behind
2. look through the crown to the base of the spine—a red ball of fire
3. looks through crown to heart chakra—pink ball of love and compassion
4. "You are a successful and confident Reiki Master / Teacher guided by Divine Love and wisdom" 3x
5. thumbs—CHO—door "I now seal this process with Divine love and wisdom" 3x
6. blessing
1. front
2. palms forward—release HY—blessing
3. move back 3 steps—hands in prayer, thank guides—open eyes—Namasté

24.1 Key to abbreviations for notes in the previous section

Abbreviation	Reiki Symbol Name
CHO	Chokurei/Chokurey
CR	Crown Chakra
DKM/D	Dai Ko Myo
Dumo	Dumo

Abbreviation	Reiki Symbol Name
FS	Fire Serpent
H	The Hara
Heart	Heart Chakra
HON	Hunshazishuneen?
HY	Hui Yin
R	Root Chakra
Ran Sai	Ran Sai
Ren So Mai	Ren So Mai
S/ SHK	Sei He Ki
SP	Solar Plexus Chakra
VB	Violet Breath

Table 1 Key to Abbreviations for Reiki Symbols

25 Reiki Waiver form

All clients are required to agree to the following release and liability waiver, which is effective for all visits.

By signing below, I acknowledge and agree that:

- <u>Insert your name</u> does not diagnose conditions, prescribe medications, or provide medical treatments.
- The sole purpose of this session/s is for relaxation or stress reduction, plus also to balance, harmonize, release and heal on all four levels of physical, mental, emotional, and spiritual.
- I understand that some bodily functions may temporarily be affected because of shifting energy within my body and I agree that this is a natural occurrence.
- I assume sole responsibility for my health and for the results of any sessions provided by <u>Insert your name</u>, which may affect my health in any way.
- Treatment/s will not replace conventional medical diagnosis or treatment. I will continue taking medication prescribed by a licensed medical physician and will continue to follow his/her instructions.
- I release <u>Insert your name</u> from all legal liability during my participation in the following Reiki treatments.
- All information received by me from <u>Insert your name</u> is accepted knowing that any action taken by me because of the information received is my complete responsibility.

Usui Tibetan Reiki Healing Energy Master / Teacher Student Manual

Insert your name & Reiki level	
Signature	Print Name
Signature of Parent or Guardian	Print name and relationship
Address—Please Print	
Date	Email Address
Phone Number	

26 Chakra Crystals

26.1 Garnet Crystal – Root Chakra

1. Stone of regeneration and stability
2. brings positive thoughts
3. excellent for manifestation and bringing abundance
4. removes negative energy from all the chakras
5. discourages disorganized growth and brings inner strength
6. stone of romantic love and passion
7. increases truth, commitment, and faith
8. reduce and / or eliminates self-sabotage (conscious or unconscious)
9. helpful in healing blood diseases, regenerating the body, metabolism, spinal and cellular disorders, blood, heart, lungs, regeneration of DNA, assimilation of minerals/vitamins, allergies, and anemia.
10. dark red

Named for the seed of the pomegranate, it is said to be good luck to be given a garnet. It is a powerfully energizing stone that protects you, bestows self-confidence and is useful in a crisis where there has been a trauma. This builds your foundation chakra and fortifies the survival instinct, bringing courage and hope. Crisis becomes a challenge under Garnet's influence and promotes mutual help. It dissolves ingrained behaviour patterns and outworn ideas that no longer serve, eliminating self-sabotaging behaviour.

26.2 Carnelian Crystal – Sacral Chakra

1. Stone of creativity, individuality, and courage.
2. Aids memory
3. assists with past life recall
4. helps to find a soul mate
5. protected from anger, jealousy, and fear
6. eases or removes sorrows

7. stabilizes energy at home,
8. helpful in healing open sores, rejuvenating tissues and cells, rheumatism, kidney stones and other kidney problems, gallstones, colds, pollen allergies and neuralgia.
9. colours orange, red, brown

The Egyptians believed this assisted the soul on its journey—they wore it to calm anger, jealousy, and envy. Carnelian is a stabilizing stone with high energy; it anchors into the present reality, the NOW, and is excellent for restoring vitality. Carnelian can cleanse other stones. It helps assist with positive life choices and is useful for overcoming abuse, including self-abuse. It helps you to trust yourself and your perceptions, overcoming negative conditioning. A stone of abundance, it motivates for success in business and any other personal areas of focus.

26.3 Citrine Crystal—Solar Plexus Chakra

1. Known as the "success" stone and the "merchant's stone"
2. promotes success and abundance (especially in business)
3. imparts generosity (receiving and giving balance)
4. enhances mental clarity, confidence, happiness, and willpower
5. brings good fortune in unexpected ways
6. alleviates depressions and self-doubt
7. brings happiness and cheer to anyone who carries it
8. diminishes mood swings and self-destructive tendencies
9. does not absorb negative energy and therefore never needs energetic clearing
10. can clear unwanted energies from environment;
11. helpful for general psychic awareness and spiritual development
12. stone for general protection removing or deflecting energies of all kinds
13. aids digestion, stomach, thyroid, heart, kidney, liver, muscles, strength, endocrine system, circulatory system, urinary system, immune system, fibromyalgia and diabetes and helps in diminishing or eliminating nightmares.
14. Colour—yellow

It absorbs, transmutes and grounds negative energy and protects the environment. It is particularly beneficial for attracting abundance. A powerful cleanse and regenerator that carries the power of the sun, this is a very beneficial stone and cleanses and re-energizes all the chakras. Energizing and highly creative, it never needs cleansing—it imparts joy to all who behold it. It reverses self-destructive behaviour and assists in acting on constructive criticism. Citrine promotes inner calm, allowing your natural wisdom to emerge and encourages emotional balance.

26.4 Rose Quartz Crystal-Heart Chakra,

1. known as the "Love stone."
2. Open heart chakra to all forms of love, self, and others
3. lowers stress
4. soothing and happy stone
5. brings gentleness, forgiveness, compassion, kindness, and tolerance.
6. Raising self-esteem and self-worth
7. emotional balancing stone
8. aids in healing emotional wounds and bringing a sense of peace and calm
9. removes fears, resentments, guilt, and anger
10. eases and aids in releasing childhood traumas
11. helpful and protective during pregnancy and with childbirth
12. helps in healing the heart, the circulatory system, fertility, headaches, kidney disease, migraines, sexual dysfunction, sinus problems, throat problems, depression, addictions, earaches, slowing signs of aging, spleen problems, fibromyalgia and maintaining an ideal weight.
13. colour—pink

A stone of unconditional love and infinite peace. Promotes receptivity to beauty in all levels—including love and self-love. An emotional healer, releasing unexpressed emotions and heartache, soothing internal pain and opening your heart so that you become receptive. If you have loved and lost, it comforts your grief. Invokes self-trust and self-worth. Excellent for trauma or crisis, it acts as a rescuer and provides reassurance and calm. Draws of negative energy strengthen empathy and sensitivity and promote necessary change.

26.5 Aquamarine Crystal — Throat Chakra

1. Known as the "stone of courage" that can bring great power
2. assists with quick intellectual response
3. brings inner peace and self-love
4. helps with shielding auras
5. brings Angels guidance and protection
6. excellent crystal for meditation
7. dispels anger and fear
8. assists with past life recall
9. beneficial in bringing about good luck
10. calms communication issues
11. being attuned to the sea. It protects travellers on water
12. helps in healing chronic fatigue, the endocrine system, eyes and eyesight, fluid retention, headaches, intestinal disorders, the nervous system, phobias, teeth and gums.
13. colour — greenish blue

Aligning all chakras, however, clears the throat chakra and opens the third eye also. A wonderful stone for meditation, it shields the aura and encourages service to humanity. Breaks self-defeating programs and leads to dynamic change. Useful also for closure on all levels, understanding underlying emotional states and interpreting how you feel. Clarifies perception as it removes extraneous thought and filters information reaching the brain.

26.6 Amethyst Crystal — Third Eye Chakra

1. known as the "meditative stone" and "calming stone"
2. provides calm, balance, patience and peace
3. equally beneficial on each of the emotional, spiritual, and physical planes
4. can assist with personal losses and grief
5. aids in emotional stability and inner strength
6. enhances flexibility and cooperation
7. can help with overcoming addictions and compulsive behaviours

8. increases spirituality and enhances intuition
9. assists in making a clear connection between the Earth plane and Source
10. helps in opening channels to telepath, past life regression as well as all "clears"
11. protects against psychic attack
12. protects against thieves and also protects travellers
13. helps healing with headaches, insomnia, arthritis, diabetes, pain relief, circulatory system issues, endocrine system, chronic fatigue, fibromyalgia, immune system, asthma, phobias, pregnancy and preventing miscarriage, menopause, PMS, and general healing
14. colour—purple

Encourages selflessness and spiritual wisdom. It also enhances metaphysical abilities and is an excellent stone to assist with meditation, dream recall, and visualization. Amethyst blocks negative environmental energies. Beneficial to the mind—calms or stimulates as necessary. It also enhances memory and improves motivation. This stone balances emotional highs and lows.

26.7 Clear Quartz—Crown Chakra

1. Known as the "Universal Crystal"
2. is a power stone
3. is the most recognized of the crystals
4. enhances energy by absorbing, storing, amplifying, balancing, focusing & transmitting
5. channels Universal energy
6. beneficial for manifesting, healing, meditation, protection and channelling
7. harmonizes and balances environment
8. energizes and strengthens healing qualities of other crystals
9. can be used to amplify healing energy and to perform diagnostic healing
10. dispels and clears away negative energy
11. enhances spiritual growth, spirituality, and wisdom
12. increases inspiration and creativity
13. assists with concentration, studying and retaining information
14. used in crystal healing to fortify and strengthen all systems of the body

15. helps in healing arthritis, bone injuries, depression, and intestinal troubles and also improves mental and physical energy, stamina, and physical strength.
16. colour—clear, white

Powerful healing and energy amplifier. It absorbs, stores, releases and regulates energy. Works at a vibrational level attuned to specific requirements of the user; it takes energy to most perfect state possible. Deep soul cleanser enhances metaphysical abilities and attunes to spiritual purpose. Quartz harmonizes all chakras, aligns the aura, and cleanses third eye chakra to enable truth to be seen in self and in situations, and signs and symbols to be recognized and understood.

27   What is the cause of a blocked chakra?

Fear, anxiety, negativity, harmful situations, emotional upsets, loss, etc., can all be causes for one or several of the chakras to become blocked or imbalanced. Negative thinking or thought patterns that can be created from any of these occurrences can create a disruption in the flow of energy through your chakras and, as a result, leave your own life force energy depleted and therefore susceptible to physical ailments or disease, emotional instability, spiritual disconnection and more.

For example, when you are thinking a negative thought, including replaying memories of past incidents that have affected you adversely or are indulging in negative self-talk or allowing yourself to remain in and be open to negative people and or situations, the "flowchart" of energy blocking might look as follows;

Negative energy from within
negative thoughts/anxiety/emotional upsets, etc.

Adversely affects the energy within the meridian's energy pathways in the body

Resulting in a decrease in life force energy being supplied to the organs—leaving them open to sickness and disease

The negative energy continues to flow through each of the chakras, creating a blockage

Due to the decrease in life force energy and blocked chakras, energy is drained away from the energy of the aura and your auric protection field is compromised, leaving you energetically open to outside negative energy.

This creates a cycle of negativity that leaves you open emotionally, physically and spiritually to continue negative thought patterns and negative outside influences.

28 How do I maintain clear and balanced chakras?

1. Sea-salt baths — Sea-salt is a natural method of detoxifying the body, as well as clearing negative energies from the aura. Regular sea-salt baths will help to maintain vitality in the body, while inducing a calm, peaceful state of being. It is also helpful to add herbs such as lavender, rosemary or rose oil to the bath. Sea salt baths should be encouraged, particularly when one is recovering from illness, surgery, or emotional distress. Sea salt is readily available at health-food stores and holistic centres.

2. Diet — Our diet is perhaps one of the most important aspects of maintaining health, yet is often the area most often overlooked when dealing with challenges or difficult emotions. During periods of stress, alcohol, caffeine, sugar and processed foods should be avoided. The first area of the body affected by stress is our immune system and a healthy diet will provide the appropriate nourishment necessary to maintain wellness.

3. Outside Air — A simple walk in nature is a POWERFUL method of cleansing the aura as well as re-energizing your entire energy field.

4. Emotions influence the vibrational level in an individual's energy field. As well, negative thoughts decrease substantially our own life force energy; the emotions of peace, love, and joy radiate with the highest energy frequencies.

5. Energy travels in circles — what is given will be received. This influences the karmic debts acquired in a lifetime. Whatever is intended for another will be experienced by you. As we understand this energy principle, we then understand that harming another actually creates harm and suffering with ourselves.

6. It is not what you do — but how you do it. A spiritual master accomplishes the most mundane of tasks in a joyful, loving manner. We are all connected. A strong, vibrant, positive, loving energy field influences all of humanity regardless of what we are physically doing. It is not the task at hand but the energy that is generated while doing it that determines the outcome.

7. Journaling — Writing about a situation and your feelings can facilitate a powerful release within the emotional body. It offers the opportunity to safely communicate to yourself and / or to another person your truths. If you are writing/venting/journalling about another person — under no circumstances are letters or emails to be sent to the person we are in conflict with. The purpose of writing is to safely release our emotions while gaining personal insight into an issue.

8. Breathing — When experiencing periods of stress or trauma, our physical body responds to these emotions by breathing very shallow half breaths. By altering our breathing patterns to deep and full breaths all the way in and exhaling all the way out, we will facilitate a release of the emotions that have contributed to our stress. Deep breathing techniques taught in yoga, Pilates, and meditation are effective tools in reducing tension and anxiety while restoring a feeling of well-being, peace, and calm.

9. Sun bath— The rays of the sun have all the seven colour energies flowing directly into your energy field, recharging and realigning each of the seven chakras. Allowing yourself to drink in the healthful rays of the sun in a responsible manner is an effective way of balancing your chakras.

10. Yoga—Specific Yoga poses are very beneficial in opening up and balancing related chakras. See 'The 7 Major Chakras section for details. Maintaining a regular yoga practice ensures balanced chakras and optimum life force energy.

11. Meditation—Personal meditation, guided meditations or walking meditations can all be useful when stimulating your chakra centres in this way and by enhancing your visualization skills and breath work. Adding your colour intentions during these exercises adds additional power to each of the chakras.

12. Crystals and gemstones—Working with crystals that align to each of the chakras on a regular basis will help to increase your energy flow and align your chakras. There are many crystals that align with each chakra, however, below are some suggestions for each; For more information on each of the crystals and more, see Crystals 101 workshops or covered more in depth in Usui Reiki Level II.

    - Root Chakra—garnet
    - Sacral Chakra—Carnelian
    - Solar Plexus Chakra—Citrine
    - Heart Chakra—Rose Quartz
    - Throat Chakra—Aquamarine
    - Third Eye Chakra—Amethyst
    - Crown Chakra—Clear Quartz

13. Aromatherapy—These essential oils are the pure essence of plants and flowers and contain healing properties. Like the crystals there are specific essences that relate to each of the 7 chakras helping to remove any blockages. A list of suggestions are as follows;

    - Root Chakra—Sandalwood
    - Sacral Chakra—ylang-ylang
    - Solar Plexus Chakra—Bergamot
    - Heart Chakra—Cedarwood
    - Throat Chakra—Patchouli
    - Third Eye Chakra—Spearmint
    - Crown Chakra—Jasmine

14. Music, Singing & Dancing—Each musical note corresponds to a colour and as well is linked to each chakra centre. Drumming, singing, dancing, tingsha bells, singing bowls, musical instruments, etc. all work together or separately to enhance the balance of your energy and chakras. See Sound Therapy and Drumming workshops and also Kirtan Music Evenings within The Clarity Centre for more detailed information on all.

15. Toning and Sounds make vibrations that can hinder our energy or balance our energy. Listen and respond to how your body and emotions react to certain sounds. Noise pollution can be very disrupting to our environment and to our energy centres. Surround yourself with sounds which resonate well with your energy—and bring joy and peace to you.

16. Solarized water—Using a clean, coloured glass bottle, fill with water and place in the sun for at least one hour. The longer the water stays in the sun, it becomes irradiated and heightens the frequency of the water taking on some of the qualities of the colour and its vibration as well as the healing properties of the sun's rays. "Solar elixirs' are one of the old-world healing sciences that have been lost but has been reborn again within the Colour Therapy and Colour Healing modalities. Drinking this water several times a day, using it to wash your vegetables or fruit, in cooking or even bathing benefits your energy and helps to clear blockages.

17. In particular, Blue Solar water represents the coolest and deepest colour of the spectrum and stands for rest, relaxation, sleep, regeneration and communication. It decreases blood pressure and heart rate and dissolves nervousness and stress providing calm. Blue solar water aids in meditation, communication and spiritual growth providing a sense of peace and balance.

Usui Tibetan Reiki Healing Energy Master / Teacher Student Manual

29 Course Descriptions and Costs

Reiki is healing energy which automatically goes to the area in your physical body or spirit where healing is most required. Reiki energy ensures that your entire spirit is in alignment by focusing on the elimination of blocks in your physical body and chakras. Your own energy is able to now move freely through your spirit and body. Reiki is totally natural and works on all levels of your life. It can relieve pain, discomfort in the physical sense and ease grief and / or anxiety as well as lack of self-confidence and insecurities. Reiki will also provide healing energy for cancer and other sickness and disease and has been found to be a proven healing modality in many other areas as well.

29.1 How will being a Reiki practitioner benefit me?

Reiki is a natural energy technique that unlocks inner flow of vital energy to restore an inner balance. After completing your Level, I am training you are able to tap into an unlimited supply of "life force energy" to improve health and enhance the quality of your life. Reiki treats the whole person including their mind, body, emotions and spirit as well as assuring a sense of peace, security and well-being. Specifically, this healing energy can assist with reducing pain, reducing stress, enhancing self-esteem and self-confidence, clearing your mind, shortening healing time and restoring energy and balance.

In this lineage, Reiki Masters are attuned to heal and teach both Usui Reiki as well as Usui/Tibetan Reiki

29.2 Reiki Level I

1. At this level, Reiki initiates will learn the following;
2. be attuned to powerful and sacred First-Degree activating initiations.
3. The Five principles of Reiki
4. The Three Pillars of Reiki
5. The history of Dr. Usui's Reiki healing
6. Gain a thorough knowledge of the Chakra system
7. Understand how energy moves through the body
8. how to release blockages and instill healing Reiki energy

9. Reiki Ethics

10. How to do a self-healing through Self Reiki

11. Become proficient in healing others in a Reiki treatment

Class is limited to 4 in-person participants in order to ensure plenty of one-on-one attention and practice time. Participants will receive their Usui Reiki Level I certificate.

Link to Manual on Amazon Kindle. eBook will download to your IOS or Android device

https://www.amazon.ca/Tibetan-Healing-Energy-Student-Manual-ebook/dp/B07J22NGYZ/ref=sr_1_1?s=digital-text&ie=UTF8&qid=1538941704&sr=1-1&keywords=Usui+Tibetan+Reiki+Healing+Energy+I+Student+Manual

29.3 Reiki Level II

Training at this level focuses on the following;

1. Level II healing symbols, their origin and precise usage
2. Receive an attunement to these symbols
3. Long distance healing with Reiki absentee healing
4. Scanning a client's energy field
5. Personal transformation and increased intuition
6. Cleansing and protection of personal energy field
7. Healing crystals and Reiki
8. Chakra balancing technique
9. Manifesting goals with Reiki
10. a complete "Reference Guide for Ailments"
11. how to use colours for healing and Reiki
12. using Marma points for healing with a Reiki session.

Usui Tibetan Reiki Healing Energy Master / Teacher Student Manual

Class is limited to 4 in-person participants to ensure one-on-one attention and practice time. Participants will receive their Usui Reiki Level II certificate.

Link to Level I Manual on Amazon Kindle—eBook will download to your IOS or Android device.

https://www.amazon.ca/Tibetan-Healing-Energy-Student-Manual-ebook/dp/B07J2134WF/ref=sr_1_1?s=digital-text&ie=UTF8&qid=1538942247&sr=1-1&keywords=Usui+Tibetan+Reiki+Healing+Energy+II+Student+Manual

29.4 Reiki Level III

Training at this level focuses on the following;

1. Usui Reiki Master Practitioner
2. Usui/Tibetan Advanced Reiki Training

At this level, Reiki initiates will learn and become proficient in the following;

1. Receive Personal Mastery Symbol for healing
2. Receive Usui/Tibetan Personal Mastery symbol
3. Attuned to all Usui/Tibetan healing symbols
4. Dr. Usui's original Healing Techniques
5. how to work with energy in the Hara
6. intensify healing treatments using the Hui Yin
7. healing with the Violet Breath
8. how to do an Etheric Cleansing
9. the Microcosmic Orbit
10. Reiki Healing Attunements
    1. Attunement for non-degree and Reiki Level I
    2. Attunement for Reiki Level II and above
    3. Self-Attunement
    4. Expansion Attunement

5. Absentee Attunement
6. Mental/emotional Attunement
7. temporarily attuning another's hands for Reiki

1. Healing Crystals
2. Crystal Power grids
3. Antahkarana Symbol
4. Receive a Usui Reiki Master Practitioner attunement
5. Receive a Usui/Tibetan Advanced Reiki Training attunement

Class is limited to 4 in-person participants to ensure one-on-one attention and practice time. Participants will receive their certificate as Usui Reiki Master Practitioner as well as Usui/Tibetan Advanced Reiki Training.

Link to Level III Manual on Amazon Kindle—eBook will download to your IOS or Android device.

https://www.amazon.ca/Tibetan-Healing-Energy-Student-Manual-ebook/dp/B07J216V1R/ref=sr_1_1?s=digital-text&ie=UTF8&qid=1538942398&sr=1-1&keywords=Usui+Tibetan+Reiki+Healing+Energy+III+Student+Manual

29.5 Usui Tibetan Reiki Master/Teacher

At this level, Reiki Masters will cover the following;

1. complete set of teaching notes and agendas
2. how to hold a healing meditation
3. numerous healing and energy meditations
4. Michael's Sword technique for healing
5. how to attune Reiki initiates to all levels of Reiki
6. Chakra invocations
7. Reiki Master Mantra
8. Reiki Ethics
9. Masters prepare an essay/project on why they wish to become a teacher of Reiki and present
10. review all levels from a teaching perspective

Usui Tibetan Reiki Healing Energy Master / Teacher Student Manual

11. practice time on how to attune others to Reiki for all levels
12. receive a digital version of all certificates, ready for print for their students
13. receive a digital version of all manuals.

    i. Usui Reiki Level I

    ii. Usui Reiki Level II

    iii. Usui Reiki Level III

    - Usui Reiki Master Practitioner
    - Usui/Tibetan Advanced Reiki Training

    iv. Usui Reiki Master/Teacher Usui/Tibetan Reiki Master

Class is usually limited to 2 in-person participants to ensure personal attention and practice time. Participants will receive their certificate as Usui Reiki Master / Teacher as well as Usui / Tibetan Reiki Master / Teacher.

30 Canadian Reiki Association

The following information is taken from The Canadian Reiki Association website at ww.reiki.ca.

If you are located in Canada, take a look. Forms and prices for membership, etc. may have changed since this manual was written.

If you are not in Canada, please refer to your national/country own Reiki Association.

30.1 Common Voice

The Canadian Reiki Association provides Reiki practitioners coast to coast with a common voice, so that we may be clearly heard when appropriate. Three newsletters per year which helps keep you up to date on social, legal, political and other issues in various areas of the country.

30.2 Affiliation

All members receive a card indicating their affiliation with the Canadian Reiki Association.

30.3 Certificate

Registered Practitioners and Registered Teachers receive a certificate attesting to their status and are entitled to use the designation RP-CRA or RT-CRA after their names.

30.4 Canadian Reiki Association Website Listing

Both registered <u>teachers</u> and <u>practitioners</u> are entitled to have their names listed on the Canadian Reiki Association website if they wish. Potential students and clients are directed to this information.

30.5 Low-Cost Professional Liability Insurance

The Canadian Reiki Association also offers the option to subscribe to our group plan for low-cost professional liability insurance. This option is available to Registered Practitioners and Registered Teachers in good standing.

30.6 Discounts

We also hope to be able to arrange member discounts with bookstores, educational providers, etc. and to bring in guest lecturers from time to time to educate our members in topics of interest.

30.7 Social Media and Newsletters

The Canadian Reiki Association is interested in ways to bring the membership together so they can get to know each other and share ideas and experiences. For those who frequent the Internet via email and website browsers, the Canadian Reiki Association has set up a Twitter and Facebook groups, which is driven by member input. The quarterly newsletter is sent to all members unless they specify otherwise. More innovations are planned in the near future.

You now have the opportunity to <u>advertise in the Canadian Reiki Association Newsletter</u> at special rates for members.

Note: Voting rights for General members exclude the right to vote for directors of the CRA. Voting rights for Registered Practitioner and Registered Teacher members have no restrictions or exclusions.

30.8 Student Members

To qualify for this level of membership, the applicant must be attuned to Reiki and have taken a Reiki Level I or Reiki First Degree class and be able to produce a copy of their Level I certificate. Student Members must sign and agree to abide by the Canadian Reiki Association Code of Ethics and the Canadian Reiki Association Disciplinary Action Policy form.

- Annual Membership Fee:

Please Note: If a Student Member wishes to continue with their training and eventually apply for Registered Practitioner Membership Level, for a six six-month period after they receive their Level I certification, they must complete the required practicum. Completion of twenty-four 24 practicum forms or a combination of practicum and C.E.U. forms, totalling twenty-four 24 hours of practice time is required. C.E.U. forms may be used when attending a Canadian Reiki Association hosted Reiki Exchange or when attending a Student Practice Night hosted by a Canadian Reiki Association Registered Teacher. Upon completion of the six 6-month practicum period and completion of twenty-four 24 hours of practice, the Student Member is eligible to apply for Registered Practitioner Membership Level.

30.9 Criteria for Registered Members

30.9.1 Registered Practitioners

To qualify as a Canadian Reiki Association Registered Practitioner, the applicant will have studied and successfully completed a minimum of Level I or first-degree Reiki class and will have completed the required practicum. The practicum requires the member to practise for at least six 6 month completing a minimum of twenty-four 24-hour practice time on "others." Practice time at Canadian Reiki Association Teacher hosted practices and Canadian Reiki Association hosted Reiki exchanges will count as 2 CEU points towards the required 24 hours. The member will submit the required and completed practicum forms and CEU forms along with their application and the applicant will sign and abide by the Canadian Reiki Association Code of Ethics and the Disciplinary Action Policy form.

If the applicant applying for this level of membership and has already graduated from Levels I, II, III and / or Master, and has been practising for a minimum of one 1 year, they must supply copies of certificates for each level of Reiki class they have graduated from and they must supply the Canadian Reiki Association with a list of 10 volunteer client case histories for a Level I graduate, 20 volunteer client case histories for Level II graduate, 30 volunteer client case histories for a Level III and / or Master graduate. They will submit the required, completed case study forms along with their application and the applicant will sign and abide by the Canadian Reiki Association Code of Ethics and the Disciplinary Action Policy form.

- Annual Membership Fee:

Please note: the number of CEUs being used towards achieving the Registered Practitioner Membership level may not be greater than 50% of the required hours i.e.: if you require 24 hours of practice time then the number of CEU's you will be allowed to use towards the 24 hours will be no greater than 12.

You must do practice sessions with at least three different clients when doing your practicum or case studies. You may not accumulate all of your hours doing sessions with the same person and you may not accumulate all of your hours with CEUs.

30.9.2 Registered Teachers

To qualify as a Canadian Reiki Association Registered Teacher, the member will have studied and successfully completed the minimum teaching requirements for the style of Reiki they studied which will consist of three or four levels of training depending on Lineage. This will not be less than three 3 levels consisting of a minimum of twenty-eight 28 hours of training in total. The member will have practised Reiki for a minimum of twice a week for a minimum of one one year from the time they received certification as a Reiki Master/Teacher. The member will read, sign and agree to abide by the Canadian Reiki Association Code of Ethics. The member will follow the Canadian Reiki Association Educational Guidelines and continually support their students by answering questions and be encouraged to host at least one student practice night per month for the purpose of issuing CEUs to student members.

Registered Teacher applicants must submit to the Canadian Reiki Association copies of their class outlines in theory and practical for review by the Canadian Reiki Association Board. Class outlines must be approved prior to Registered Membership status being granted. Class outlines may be submitted in pdf to membership@reiki.ca or mailed to the CRA. They must also visibly display their Canadian Reiki Association designation and their Canadian Reiki Association Registration number on every certificate they issue to their students.

Example: RT-054 will be displayed beside the Teacher's name.

- Annual Membership Fee:

Please note: Registered Teacher applicants who are not Canadian Reiki Association Registered Practitioners and are applying to be a Canadian Reiki Association Registered Teacher "only," you must also abide by the Canadian Reiki Association Practitioner Criteria and supply the Canadian Reiki Association with 30 volunteer client case histories along with all other requested forms.

30.10 Referrals for RP/RT-CRA

Upon request, the Canadian Reiki Association will give to the public, the names of Registered Practitioners/Teachers who meet the above criteria, providing the member has given permission. In order to activate this process, a Canadian Reiki Association Registered member must fill out and sign the referral section at the bottom of the Code of Ethics and indicate their preferences for the location for treating the client and / or teaching the client.

31 Listings for RP/RT-CRA at the Canadian Reiki Association Internet Page

Registered Practitioners/Teachers meeting the above criteria may list their name, location, phone, email and website at the Canadian Reiki Association Registered Teachers page provided they fill out the related permission form available at the website or from the Canadian Reiki Association.

32 I believe…

- I believe the Divine lives within each one of us
- I believe we can heal ourselves
- I believe we can help others to awaken their own healing power.
- I believe in pure joy
- I believe bliss lies in simplicity
- I believe the answer to every issue becomes available when you open your mind to the possibility.
- I believe that learning to live in the present moment is the key to uncovering "the power of self."
- I believe laughter is powerful in its healing capacity
- I believe compassion and love provide a gateway and safe passage through anger and fear to a new landscape of greater understanding and peace.
- I believe we set down our own paths before we come here on this journey and feel a comfortable fit as we unite with people and situations that allow us to reach our milestones.
- I believe we are all "human connectors" between Mother Earth and the Divine. I believe wherever we have walked we leave a footprint of the unity—a column of light in our path to shine for others.
- I believe every day that I believe creates more to believe in.
- I believe in the power of one.
- I believe in the power of many—working together as one.
- I boliovo in Bolioving.

www.ingramcontent.com/pod-product-compliance
Lightning Source LLC
Chambersburg PA
CBHW041545220426
43665CB00002B/40